HERBS

For Flavor, Health, and Natural Beauty

written by
Jim Rude & Jena Carlin

food styling by
Jim Rude
www.rudeonfood.com

photography by
Jena Carlin
www.jenacarlincreative.com

www.littlerustedladle.com

HERBS

For Flavor, Health, and Natural Beauty

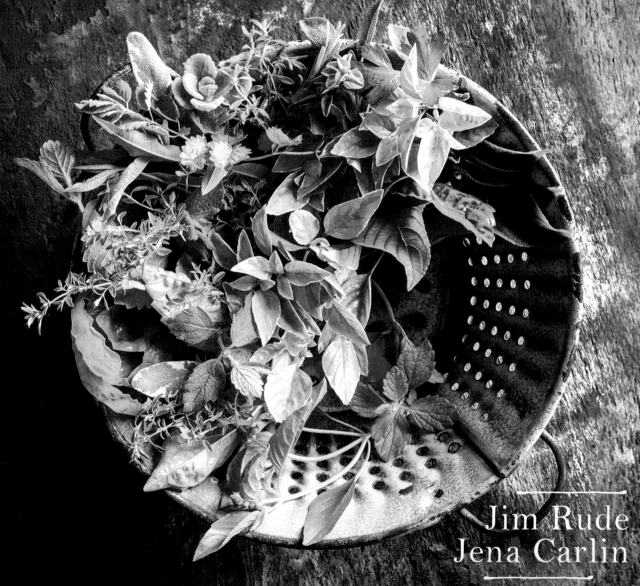

Jim Rude
Jena Carlin

HOBBLE CREEK PRESS | AN IMPRINT OF CEDAR FORT, INC. | SPRINGVILLE, UTAH

ISBN 13: 978-1-4621-1972-1

Published by Hobble Creek Press, an imprint of Cedar Fort, Inc.
2373 W. 700 S., Springville, UT 84663
Distributed by Cedar Fort, Inc., www.cedarfort.com

LIBRARY OF CONGRESS CATALOGING-IN-PUBLICATION DATA

Names: Rude, Jim, 1966- author. | Carlin, Jena, 1984- author.
Title: Herbs for Flavor, Health, and Natural Beauty / Jim Rude and Jena
 Carlin.
Description: Springville, Utah : Hobble Creek Press, an imprint of Cedar
 Fort, Inc., [2017] | Includes bibliographical references and index.
Identifiers: LCCN 2016054433 | ISBN 9781462119721 (hardback : acid-free paper)
Subjects: LCSH: Cooking (Herbs) | Herbs--Therapeutic use. | LCGFT: Cookbooks.
Classification: LCC TX819.H4 R84 2017 | DDC 641.6/57--dc23
LC record available at https://lccn.loc.gov/2016054433

Cover and page design by Priscilla Chaves
Cover design © 2017 Cedar Fort, Inc.
Photography by Jena Carlin
Food Styling by Jim Rude
Edited by Jessica Romrell & Erica Myers

Printed in the United States of America

10 9 8 7 6 5 4 3 2 1

Printed on acid-free paper

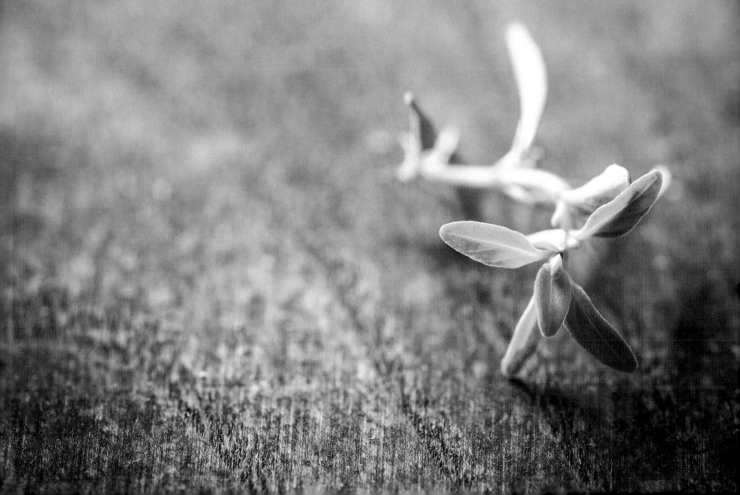

Dedicated to:

*Our parents who raised and loved us, our friends
and family who are always there for us, the many
farmers in the world who provide for us, and our
creator, who has made everything possible.*

Contents

Acknowledgments

Writing about herbs was a natural choice for my first cookbook. I have very fond childhood memories of my parents growing all varieties of fresh herbs, flowers, fruits, and vegetables in our backyard garden. My mom would have me smell and taste the different herbs, patiently taking time to explain what they were. As I grew up, graduated from culinary school, and worked as a chef, those herbs became the foundation of my cooking style. Later, as my career evolved to food styling, I began growing my own herbs that ultimately would be used in photographs of food seen all over the world.

As it is almost a year to the day after my mom's passing, it is only fitting that I dedicate this book to her and our shared love for herbs. *Herbs for Flavor, Health, and Natural Beauty* is my loving gratitude to my mother, Phyllis, for instilling that passion in me. I'd also like to thank my dad, Patrick, who showed me how to cook by taste and feel, rather than by simply following recipes.

Since food transcends from generation to generation, I'd like to thank my wonderful children, Logan and Kennedy. Without you, my life would have no meaning. If I give you nothing else, I wish to hand down my love of food. It connects people like nothing else on this planet. Embrace it and always cook with love and live to cook.

Thank you to my dear Judi, whose encouraging words and support kept me going from start to finish. I'd also like to thank my friends, family, and neighbors, especially my best friends Chris, Dana, and Doug and Co. for tasting and testing the many culinary concoctions I've created and made them eat over the years.

Last, but not least, this book is not possible without my blogging partner and dear friend, Jena Carlin. Your energy, creativity, and talent amaze me every time I work with you. Working on our blog and on this book has re-energized my passion for food in ways I can't describe. Thank you.

–JIM RUDE

Acknowledgments

Growing up, I would spend hours with my mother creating all sorts of crafts: wreaths, stained glass, candle making, and scrapbooking, to name a few. I loved the smell of our sun porch where we worked. The scent of dried botanicals and hot glue filled the air. Photography was also a big hobby of ours. By the time I was fourteen, I knew I wanted to be a photographer. Spending time with my mother making anything and everything are my favorite memories with her.

That is why I would like to dedicate this book to my mother, Wanda Weiler, for spending time with me creating. I would also like to thank my father, Alan Weiler, for being an extraordinary example of work ethic, and for raising me on a farm where I grew to appreciate where my food comes from. Thank you to my husband, Brandon, and our ever-growing family—which includes, but is not limited to, my son, Austin, and Baby Carlin #2—for your support and enriching my life beyond words. Lastly, thank you to Jim Rude for saying yes to starting Little Rusted Ladle with me. I am blessed to be working with such a talented and seasoned food stylist. You make my job easier and I have enjoyed eating everything you made for this book.

–JENA CARLIN

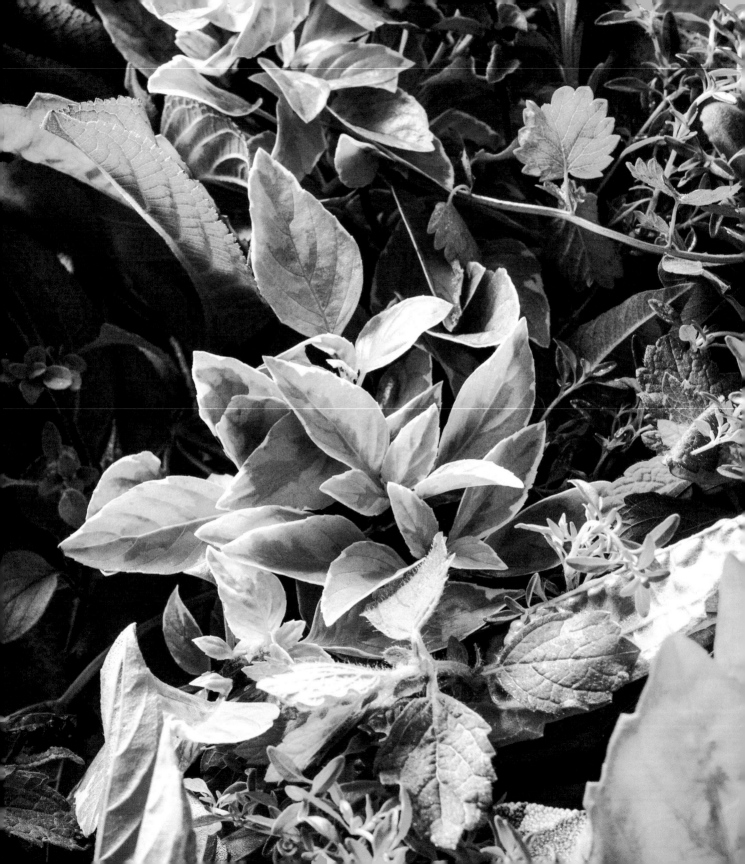

Introduction

Less than a year ago, Jena and I were approached to write a cookbook. It would be our first one, so we weren't quite sure which direction to take it. Since Little Rusted Ladle is about all things yummy, it could go just about anywhere—healthy, natural, decadent, or perhaps themed by ingredients, holidays, or parties.

In the end, the option that made the most sense to us was probably the simplest: a book about herbs in all their glory. Not just about cooking with herbs, but creating with them, in and out of the kitchen. I think for both of us, herbs take us on a journey back to our childhood and the memories we shared with our moms who lovingly taught us so much about gardening, cooking, and creating beautiful things. Today, we enjoy making similar memories with our own children.

Jena and I strongly appreciate the beauty of nature. To us, the simplicity of herbs is natural perfection: The graceful elegance of a simple leaf. The way herbs appeal to every one of our senses. They are so important, though we rarely even think about them. Herbs give us nourishment, they appeal to us visually, they make us feel better, and they help us in ways we may never really understand.

Herbs also have the ability to do what other foods like fruits, vegetables, or grains lack. They keep growing, providing the same wonders over and over again. A single lemon, for example, takes months to grow, only to be picked once, its fruit enjoyed, then discarded. Lemon balm, however, grows bigger the more you harvest it, and every time you run your hands across its leaves, you are rewarded with the smell of fresh lemons.

Similarly, once you pick a green onion, it's gone. You have to plant more, whereas chives keep growing even after harvesting, and they produce beautiful flowers that are edible as well. The same goes for so many other herbs. When was the last time you rubbed a piece of lettuce and it smelled like licorice, or munched on celery that actually tasted like a peppery radish? Herbs give and keep giving and encourage you to harvest them often so that they can grow in size. It's a perfect relationship. We harvest them, enjoying all they have to offer, which also encourages their growth.

The oils and healing properties of herbs are legendary. Many of the man-made pharmaceuticals, perfumes, and healthcare products we use every day wouldn't be possible without herbs. Can you turn a tomato into a wreath, a perfume, a soap, or lip balm while also enjoying its flavor in a recipe? You can with many herbs. This book is about the flavor, health, and natural beauty of herbs.

Jena and I hope you enjoy our concept of what an herb cookbook should look like. Herbs are a beautiful gift given to us by Mother Nature. We celebrate all they give us, and we hope you appreciate them as much as we do.

Enjoy!

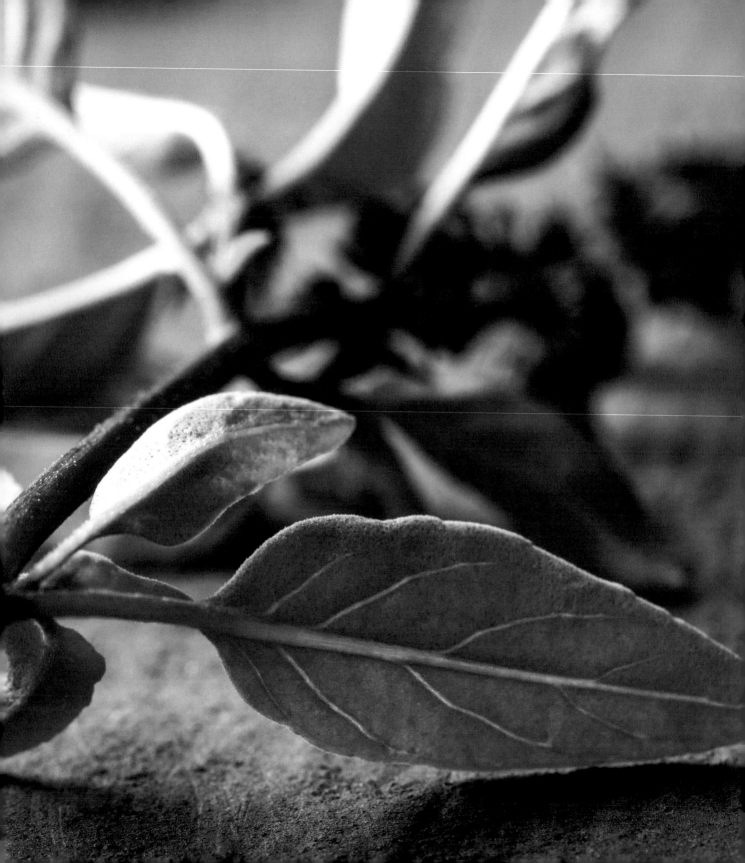

Chapter 1:
BASIL

*T*he sweet yet spicy licorice flavors of basil have been transforming recipes from drab and flavorless to legendary for literally thousands of years. Basil has been linked to many ancient remedies and culinary dishes in Italy, Thailand, India, and Greece, where its name originated as "basilikon phuton." or "royal plant." Thank goodness we shortened it to basil. It is also the victim of historic imagination. It was once thought that basil could cause scorpions to grow in the brain. I'm pretty sure its reputation would have suffered greatly if that were true. Many cultures depend on basil as a major flavoring in their cuisines. Can you imagine classic pesto without basil? How about a caprese salad or bruschetta? No thank you.

Basil is without a doubt one of the most popular herbs in the kitchen. Simply rubbing a leaf or two between your fingers, then breathing in the wonderful aroma of the oils being released will put a smile on your face. Add those same leaves to a tart, soup, or even chocolate dessert or ice cream float, and that smile will transfer to your taste buds.

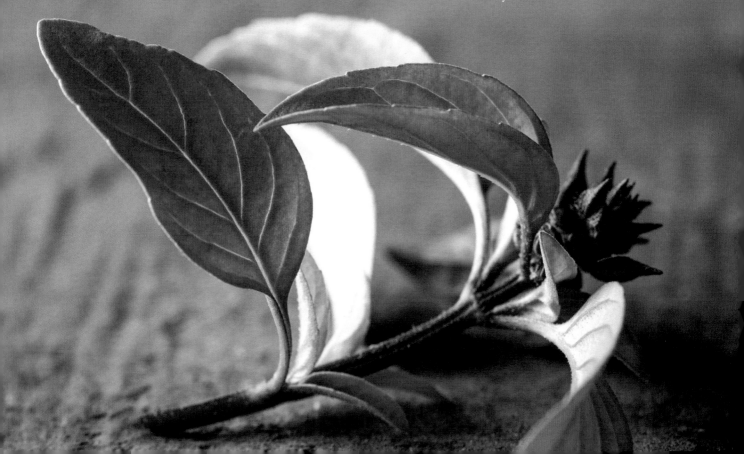

APRICOT & BASIL GALETTE

This galette is a great way to enjoy fresh apricots when they are in season. Fresh basil takes this appetizer to a new level, and the smokey bacon and pine nuts are a perfect final touch.

4 whole fresh apricots, halved

2 tsp. vegetable oil

¼ cup ricotta cheese

¼ cup mascarpone cheese

2 Tbsp. fresh basil, finely chopped, divided

1 refrigerated 9-inch piecrust

2 tsp. whole wheat flour

1 Tbsp. simple syrup

1 slice smoked bacon, cooked, chopped

8–10 small fresh basil leaves

1 Tbsp. pine nuts, toasted

1. Lightly brush apricot halves with vegetable oil. Grill cut side down on a very hot grill for 30–45 seconds or until slightly soft. Remove apricots with a flat spatula. Let cool, then cut into slices.

2. IN A SMALL BOWL, stir together ricotta cheese, mascarpone cheese, and basil until smooth. Set aside.

3. Unroll pie dough, and sprinkle 1 teaspoon of flour on each side.

4. Spoon reserved cheese mixture into center of piecrust and spread mixture to within two inches of the edge. Place apricot slices overlapping on top of the cheese. Brush apricots with honey. Fold edges over filling. Bake at 375 degrees for 20–25 minutes or until crust is golden brown. Remove from oven and let cool to room temperature. Sprinkle bacon, pine nuts, and basil leaves on top. Serve.

SERVINGS: 4 | SOURCE: Little Rusted Ladle

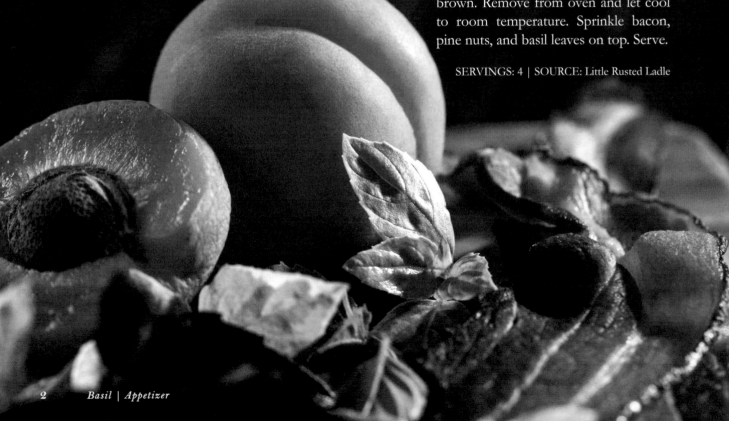

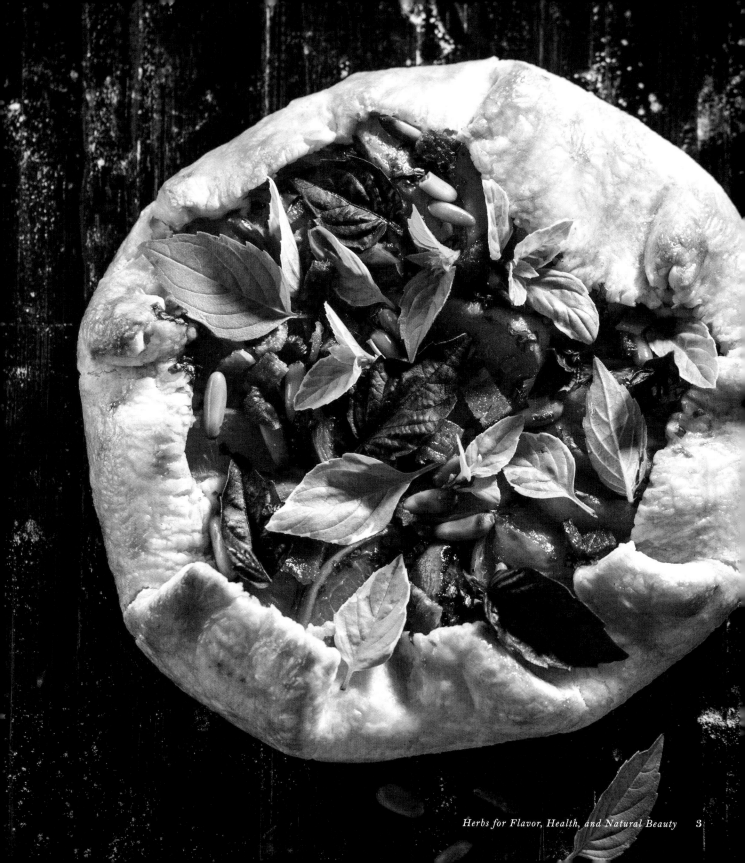

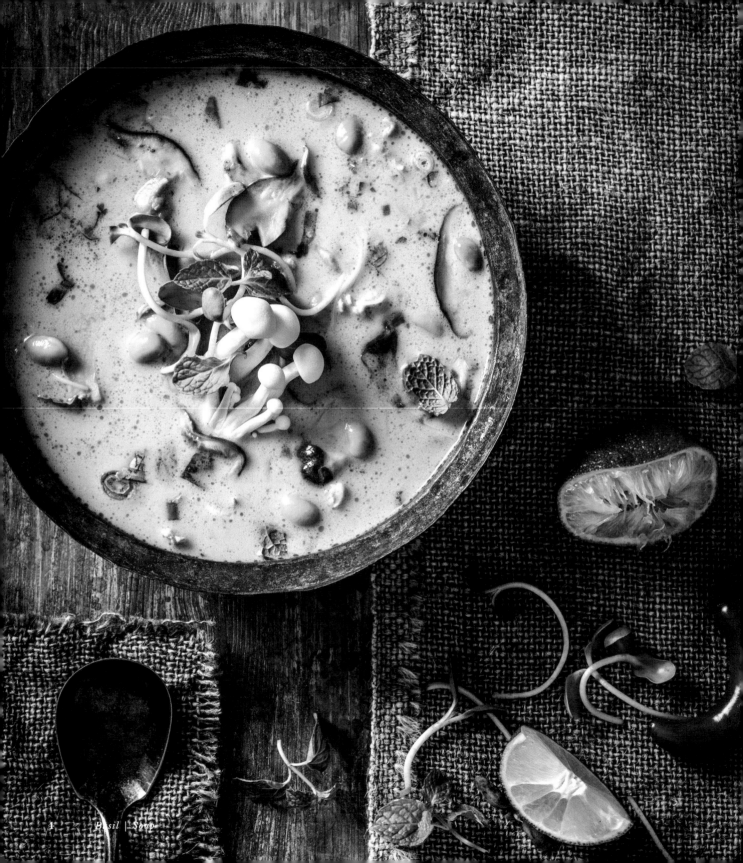

CURRY COCONUT CHICKEN SOUP

The exotic flavors of curry, coconut, lime juice, mint, basil, and hot peppers will explode in your mouth making you wish you were in tropical Thailand.

¼ cup chopped onion

1 tsp. green curry paste

1 tsp. red curry paste

1 garlic cloves, minced

1 tsp. fresh ginger, minced

½ cup yellow bell pepper, diced

½ cup shiitake mushrooms, sliced

1 Tbsp. vegetable oil

3 cups reduced sodium chicken broth

2 boneless, skinless chicken thighs

1¼ cups coconut milk

1 tsp. curry powder

1 Tbsp. light brown sugar

¼ tsp. crushed red pepper flakes

1 whole green onions, thinly sliced

1 Tbsp. fresh cilantro, chopped

serrano pepper slices

¼ cup frozen edamame, thawed

¼ cup sunflower sprouts, optional

2 Tbsp. fresh basil leaves, chopped

1 Tbsp. fresh mint leaves

¼ cup enoki mushrooms, optional

4 slices lime

1. IN A LARGE STOCKPOT OR DUTCH OVEN, sauté onion, curry paste, garlic, ginger, bell pepper, and shiitake mushrooms in oil over medium heat until softened.

2. Add chicken broth and bring to a simmer. Add chicken thighs. Simmer on low for 15–20 minutes or until chicken is cooked through. Remove chicken with a pair of tongs, and set aside until cool enough to handle. Pull chicken into pieces, and set aside.

3. Add coconut milk, curry powder, brown sugar, and red pepper flakes to soup. Simmer until coconut milk has melted completely. Add chicken to soup and simmer for 15 minutes.

4. Ladle into bowls, and serve topped with green onions, cilantro, serrano pepper slices, edamame, sunflower sprouts, basil, mint leaves, enoki mushrooms, and lime.

SERVINGS: 4 | SOURCE: Little Rusted Ladle

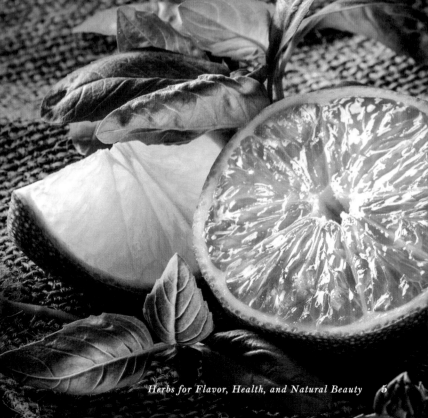

FRESH SWEET CORN
& BLUEBERRY SALAD

Sweet corn and blueberries are a match made in heaven. Add basil and mint to the equation and heaven just got better. For a refreshing summer snack, omit the arugula and serve the mixture as a salsa with tortilla chips.

4 ears sweet corn (2 cups), kernels removed

4 cups arugula, washed

1 cup blueberries

1 (4 oz.) can diced green chiles, drained

¼ cup shelled pistachios, toasted

2 Tbsp. fresh basil leaves, chopped

1 Tbsp. fresh mint leaves, chopped

¼ cup light olive oil

2 Tbsp. fresh lime juice

1 Tbsp. honey

Salt & pepper to taste

1. Combine first seven ingredients in a medium size bowl.

2. IN A SMALL BOWL, whisk together olive oil, lime juice, and honey.

3. Add dressing mixture to salad mixture and toss to coat. Serve.

SERVINGS: 4 | SOURCE: Little Rusted Ladle

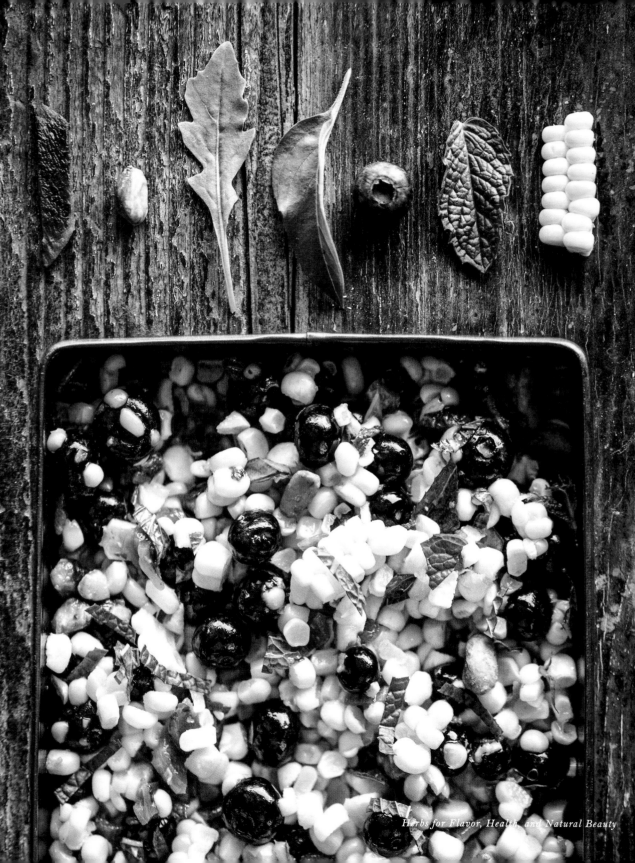

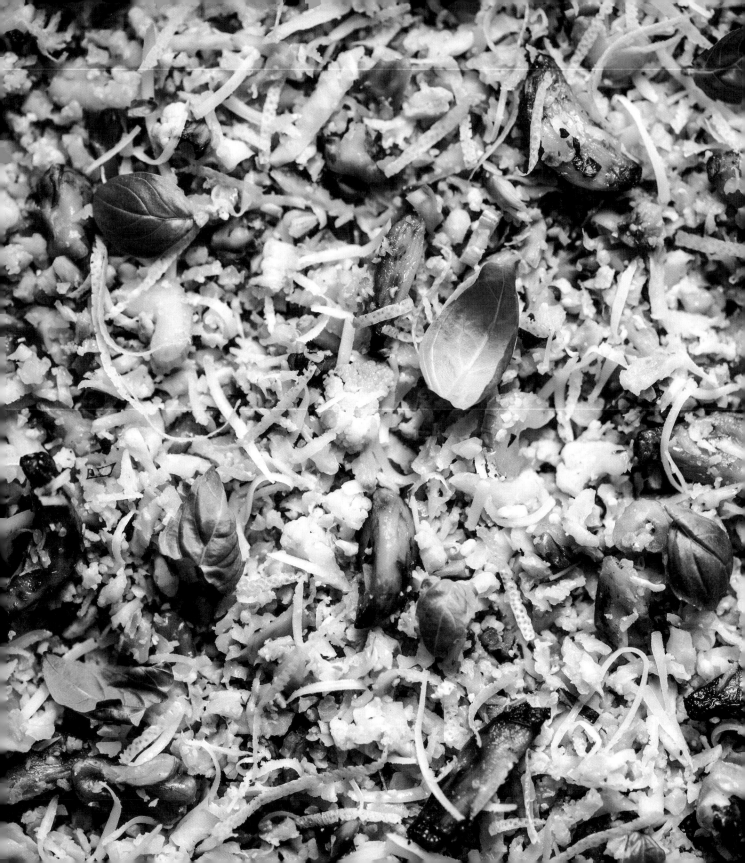

ROASTED CAULIFLOWER RICE WITH BASIL

Finely chopped cauliflower is a healthy alternative to white rice. Roasted garlic, celery, walnuts, and romanesco add color and crunch, while the basil, lemon, and parmesan cheese help transform this often overlooked vegetable from drab to glam. If romanesco is not available, simply increase the amount of cauliflower.

1. Preheat oven to 400 degrees. Lightly coat garlic cloves with a small amount of the coconut oil and place on a sheet pan lined with nonstick foil or spray pan with nonstick spray. Roast for 20 minutes. Remove pan from oven.

2. IN A LARGE BOWL, combine cauliflower and next four ingredients with remaining oil. Toss to coat. Transfer mixture to the sheet pan with garlic. Roast for 20–25 minutes or until lightly browned in areas.

3. Remove pan from oven and top with lemon zest and parmesan cheese. Transfer mixture to a serving bowl and gently toss with a serving spoon. Season to taste with salt and pepper. Serve.

SERVINGS: 4 | SOURCE: Little Rusted Ladle

12 garlic cloves, peeled

2 Tbsp. coconut oil, melted

4 cups cauliflower florets, finely chopped

½ cup romanesco, finely chopped, optional

1 stalk celery, thinly sliced

½ cup walnut pieces

½ cup small basil leaves

1 Tbsp. grated lemon zest

¼ cup parmesan cheese, shredded, optional

Salt and pepper to taste

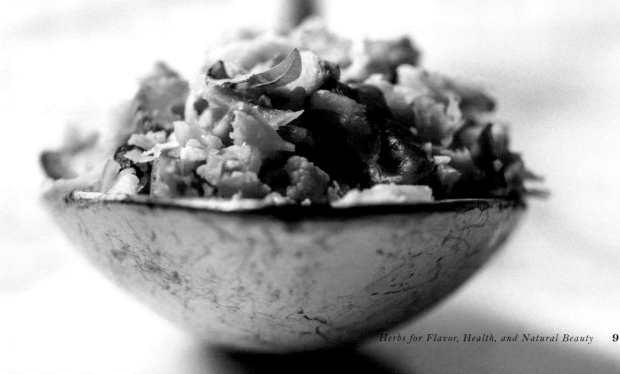

Pesto is a staple in every Italian kitchen. This recipe embraces that tradition, then adds a little kick by adding some green chiles and lime juice.

1. Preheat oven to 450 degrees. Rub peppers with a small amount of olive oil. Roast in oven for 20–25 minutes. Remove from oven and cool completely. Remove skins, then split in half lengthwise. Discard seeds and stems. Place peppers in a food processor.

2. Add basil, olive oil, parmesan cheese, and lime juice to food processor with peppers. Process for 30 seconds or until mixture is smooth, scraping down sides once or twice if needed. Transfer to a large bowl and set aside.

3. Cook pasta according to directions. Drain pasta, then add to bowl with prepared pesto. Season to taste with salt and pepper. Divide pasta evenly between four shallow bowls. Top each with halved tomatoes, prosciutto, parmesan shavings, and fresh basil leaves. Serve.

SERVINGS: 4
SOURCE: Little Rusted Ladle

FETTUCCINE WITH TRIPLE BASIL JALAPEÑO PESTO

5 Jalapeño peppers

2 cups fresh basil leaves, packed

½ cup extra virgin olive oil

¼ cup parmesan cheese, grated

1 Tbsp. fresh lime juice

18 oz. fettucine

Salt and pepper to taste

12 whole grape tomatoes, halved

4 slices prosciutto, halved lengthwise

Parmesan cheese shavings, for garnish

Fresh basil leaves, for garnish

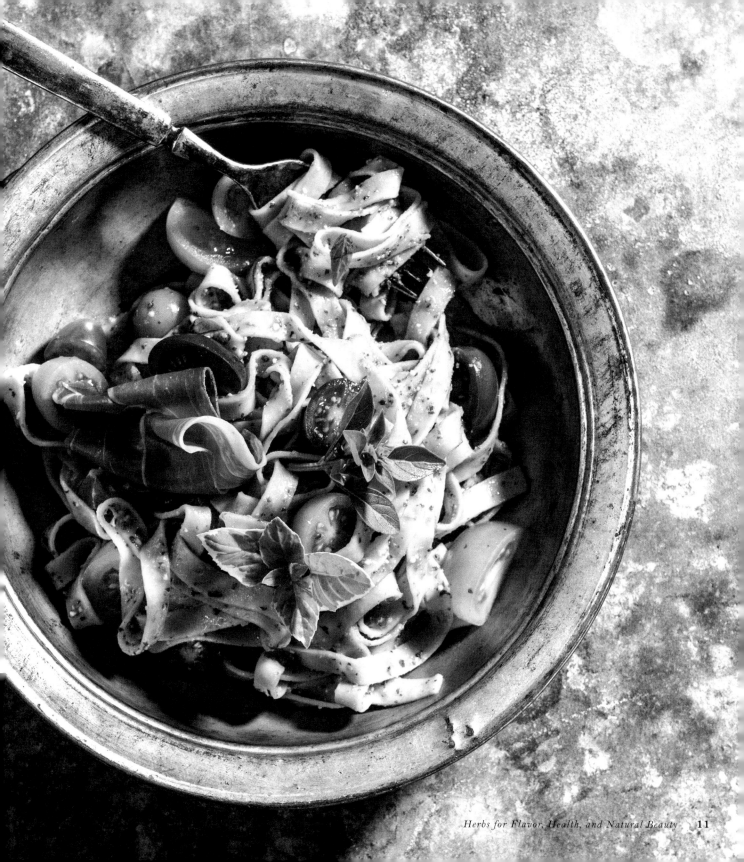

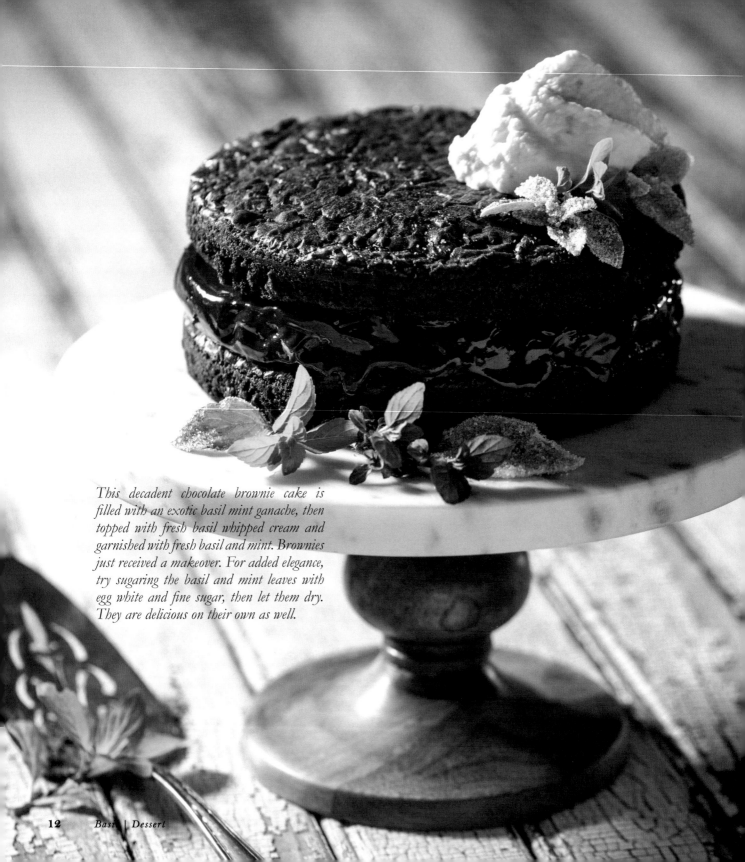

This decadent chocolate brownie cake is filled with an exotic basil mint ganache, then topped with fresh basil whipped cream and garnished with fresh basil and mint. Brownies just received a makeover. For added elegance, try sugaring the basil and mint leaves with egg white and fine sugar, then let them dry. They are delicious on their own as well.

CHOCOLATE BASIL BROWNIE TORTE WITH BASIL CREAM

Cocoa powder

1 (19.9–oz.) pkg. fudge brownie mix

½ cup coconut oil

2 large eggs, beaten

¼ cup water

1 cup heavy cream, divided

½ cup fresh basil leaves, divided

¼ cup fresh chocolate mint leaves, divided

¾ cup semisweet chocolate chips

1 Tbsp. powdered sugar

1 tsp. pure vanilla extract

4–6 sprigs fresh basil, for garnish, optional

4–6 sprigs fresh mint, for garnish, optional

1. Preheat oven to 350 degrees. Line the bottoms of two 6-inch cake pans with nonstick foil or parchment paper circles cut to fit bottom of pan. Spray sides with nonstick spray, then dust sides with cocoa powder. Set pans aside while making batter.

2. FOR BROWNIE LAYERS, in a large mixing bowl, combine brownie mix, coconut oil, eggs, and water. Fill pans halfway with batter. Pour remaining batter into muffin tins or reserve for another use. Bake brownie cakes according to the directions on the package or until a toothpick inserted in the center comes out clean. Transfer to a cooling rack and let cool completely, then cover and refrigerate until ready to assemble.

3. FOR GANACHE FILLING, in a medium saucepan, bring heavy cream to a simmer over medium-low heat. Chop basil and mint leaves, and put 1 tablespoon of each herb in a small bowl. Set aside to use for the cream. Stir the remaining basil and mint leaves into the hot cream. Take pan off the heat and let herbs steep in the cream for ten minutes. Pour cream through a strainer, reserving cream. Discard herbs. Place chocolate chips in a heatproof bowl. Slowly whisk ½ cup of the strained cream into chocolate chips until mixture is smooth and all chocolate has melted. Refrigerate remaining cream to use for the basil cream. Cover and refrigerate ganache mixture until firm (about 45 minutes).

4. FOR BASIL CREAM, combine reserved cream and powdered sugar in a small bowl. Beat with a hand mixer on medium speed until soft peaks form. Stir in vanilla and reserved chopped basil and mint. Cover and refrigerate until ready to serve.

5. TO ASSEMBLE, remove brownie cakes by running a knife around the inside edge of pan. Turn pan upside down over a sheet of parchment paper or plastic wrap and remove the cake from the pan. Repeat with remaining cake. Place one cake on a serving plate. Spread cold ganache mixture over the top of one cake. Top with remaining cake. Spoon dollops of basil cream on top of cake and garnish with fresh basil and mint sprigs.

SERVINGS: 4 | SOURCE: Little Rusted Ladle

BERRY BASIL FLOATS

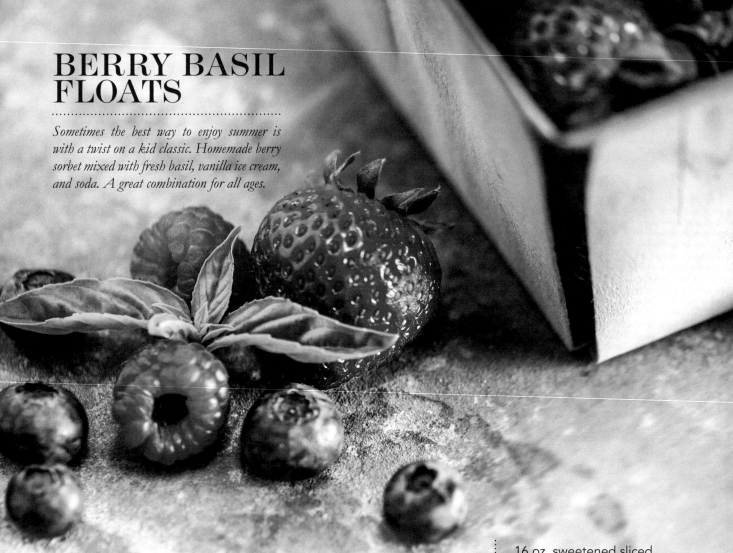

Sometimes the best way to enjoy summer is with a twist on a kid classic. Homemade berry sorbet mixed with fresh basil, vanilla ice cream, and soda. A great combination for all ages.

1. FOR BASIL BERRY SORBET, puree strawberries, raspberries, and basil leaves in a blender until smooth. Transfer to a medium bowl. Strain mixture through a fine strainer. There should be about 2 cups. Freeze until solid, about two hours. If desired, run the mixture through an ice cream machine to make it smoother when scooping.

2. FOR BASIL BERRY FLOAT, remove frozen berry mixture and ice cream from freezer and let sit at room temperature for 15 minutes. Spoon four large spoonfuls of berry mixture into four tall collins glasses, then four large spoonfuls of ice cream. Repeat once more. Top with lemon-lime soda, fresh basil sprig, and a strawberry. Serve immediately.

SERVINGS: 4 | SOURCE: Little Rusted Ladle

16 oz. sweetened sliced strawberries, thawed

12 oz. frozen raspberries, thawed

2 cups fresh basil leaves, loosely packed

2 cups vanilla ice cream

2 cups lemon-lime soda, chilled

Fresh basil sprig and strawberries, for garnish, optional

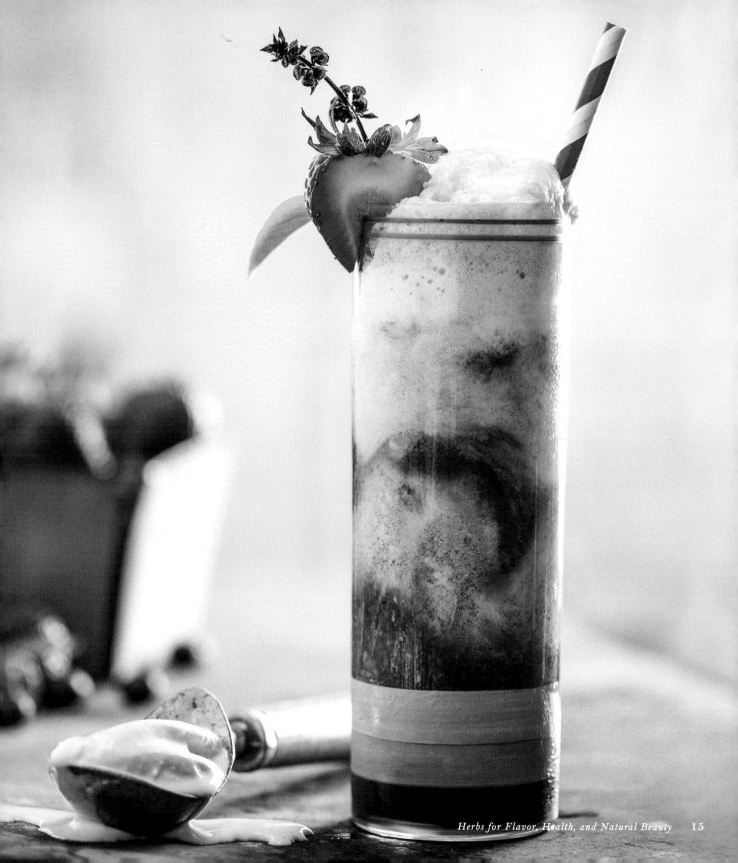

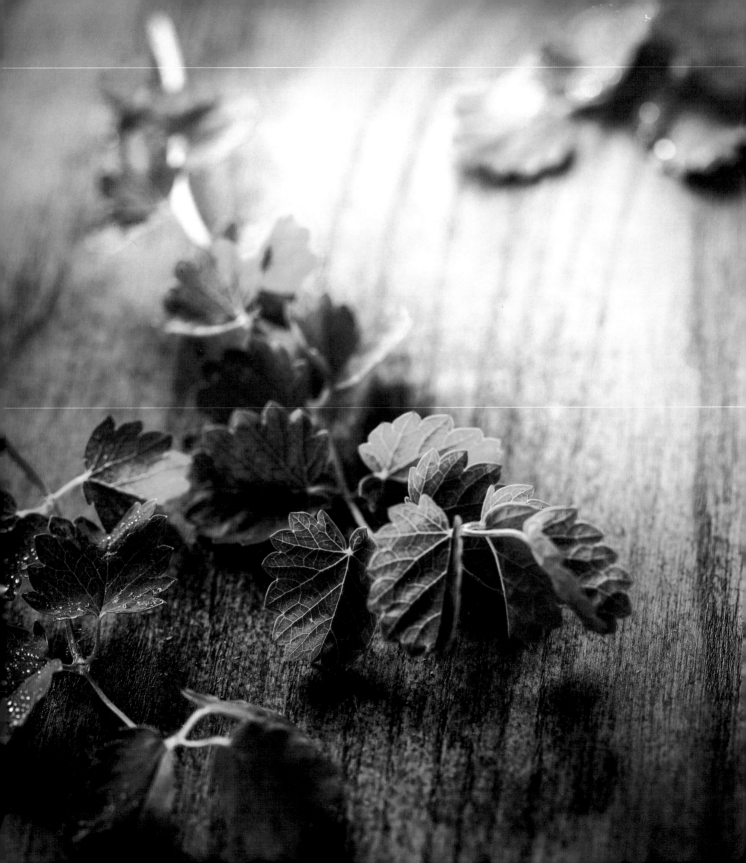

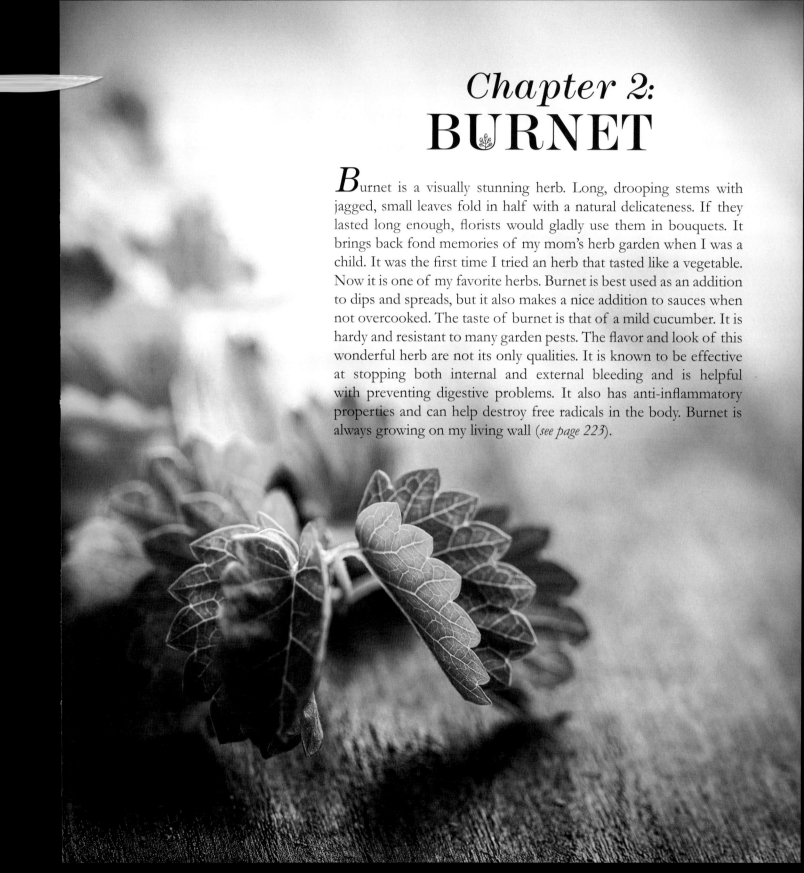

Chapter 2:
BURNET

*B*urnet is a visually stunning herb. Long, drooping stems with jagged, small leaves fold in half with a natural delicateness. If they lasted long enough, florists would gladly use them in bouquets. It brings back fond memories of my mom's herb garden when I was a child. It was the first time I tried an herb that tasted like a vegetable. Now it is one of my favorite herbs. Burnet is best used as an addition to dips and spreads, but it also makes a nice addition to sauces when not overcooked. The taste of burnet is that of a mild cucumber. It is hardy and resistant to many garden pests. The flavor and look of this wonderful herb are not its only qualities. It is known to be effective at stopping both internal and external bleeding and is helpful with preventing digestive problems. It also has anti-inflammatory properties and can help destroy free radicals in the body. Burnet is always growing on my living wall (*see page 223*).

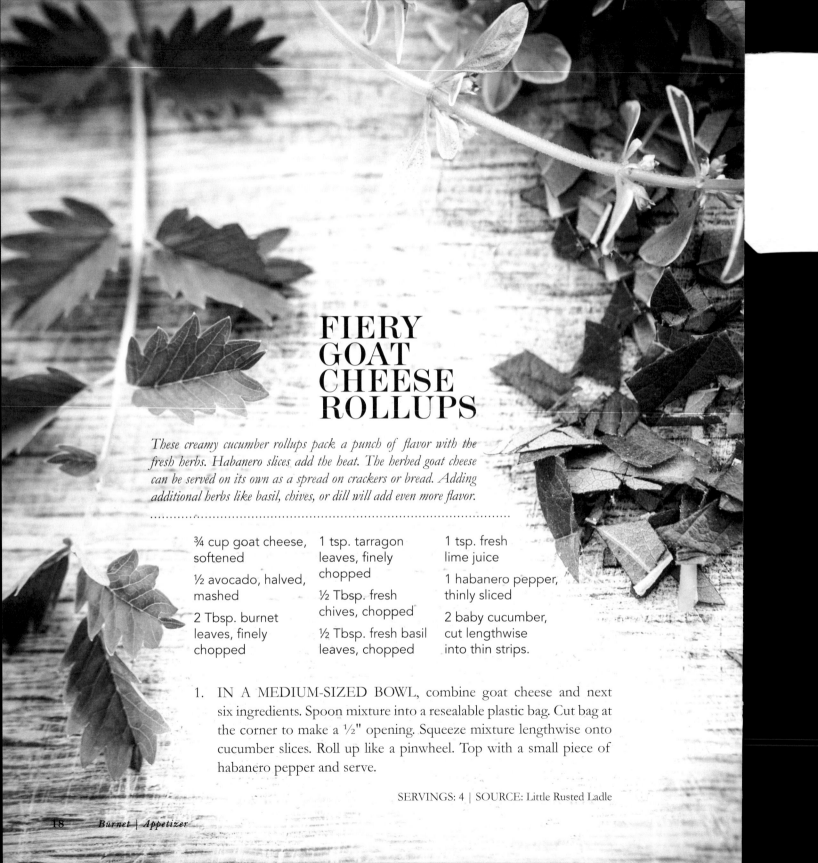

FIERY GOAT CHEESE ROLLUPS

These creamy cucumber rollups pack a punch of flavor with the fresh herbs. Habanero slices add the heat. The herbed goat cheese can be served on its own as a spread on crackers or bread. Adding additional herbs like basil, chives, or dill will add even more flavor.

¾ cup goat cheese, softened

½ avocado, halved, mashed

2 Tbsp. burnet leaves, finely chopped

1 tsp. tarragon leaves, finely chopped

½ Tbsp. fresh chives, chopped

½ Tbsp. fresh basil leaves, chopped

1 tsp. fresh lime juice

1 habanero pepper, thinly sliced

2 baby cucumber, cut lengthwise into thin strips.

1. IN A MEDIUM-SIZED BOWL, combine goat cheese and next six ingredients. Spoon mixture into a resealable plastic bag. Cut bag at the corner to make a ½" opening. Squeeze mixture lengthwise onto cucumber slices. Roll up like a pinwheel. Top with a small piece of habanero pepper and serve.

SERVINGS: 4 | SOURCE: Little Rusted Ladle

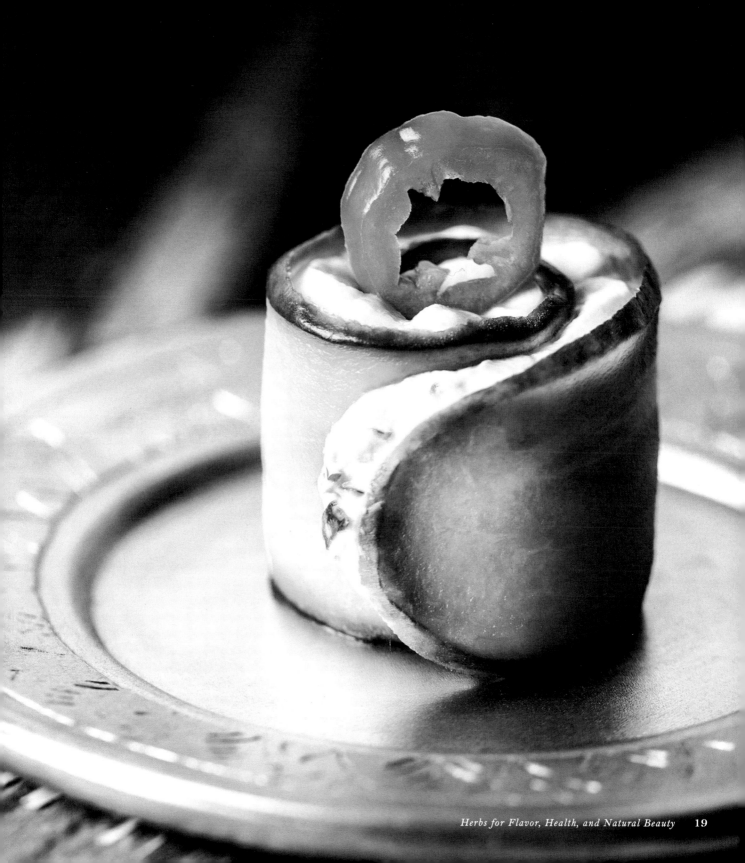

Herbs for Flavor, Health, and Natural Beauty   19

The taste of fresh tomatoes at the peak of summer is something to remember. This traditional chilled tomato soup utilizes the flavors of three different kinds of tomatoes as well as peppers and zucchini to give it exceptional fresh flavor. Fresh burnet leaves add a mild cucumber taste that brings it all together. For a nice smokey flavor, grill the peppers and zucchini before cubing them.

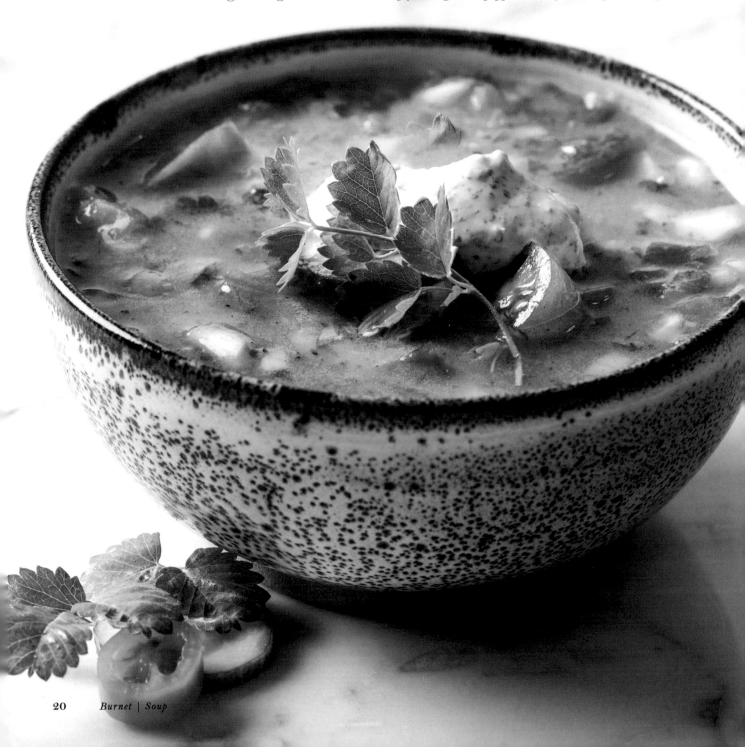

GAZPACHO WITH BURNET CREMA

4 cups yellow cherry tomatoes

3 garlic cloves, peeled

1 tsp. kosher salt

½ tsp. fresh ground black pepper

½ cup cubed orange bell pepper

½ cup cubed red bell pepper

½ cup chopped poblano pepper

½ cup chopped zucchini

2 medium tomatillos, chopped

1 cup quartered grape tomatoes, assorted colors

Salt and pepper to taste

½ cup mexican crema or sour cream

1 cup burnet leaves, loosely packed

½ tsp. kosher salt

1. FOR YELLOW TOMATO GAZPACHO, combine yellow cherry tomatoes and next three ingredients in a food processor. Process until smooth. Strain mixture through a fine mesh strainer into a large bowl, removing as much of the seeds and skins as possible. Discard skins and seeds. Set aside.

2. Place peppers, zucchini, and tomatillos in a baking dish. Toss with oil. Broil in oven on high for 7–10 minutes or until slightly charred. Remove from oven and let cool. Refrigerate for 30 minutes. Transfer mixture to food processor and pulse 3–4 times until roughly chopped. Add mixture to bowl of strained tomato juice. Stir in quartered grape tomatoes. Season gazpacho to taste with salt and pepper. Refrigerate until ready to serve.

3. FOR BURNET CREMA, combine crema or sour cream in a food processor with burnet leaves and kosher salt. Process until smooth. Transfer to a small dish and refrigerate until ready to serve.

4. TO SERVE, ladle cold gazpacho into bowls. Top with a dollop of burnet cream and garnish with fresh burnet leaves. Serve.

SERVINGS: 4 | SOURCE: Little Rusted Ladle

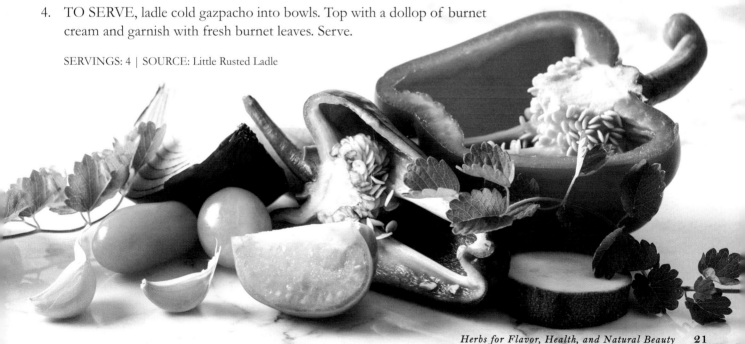

BURNET SLAW WITH CHAMPAGNE GUAVA VINAIGRETTE

Nappa cabbage is the canvas for this light and refreshing slaw recipe. Burnet is the star, with flavors of basil and nasturtium following close behind. Guava nectar, which can be found in the Hispanic section of most grocery stores, works well in a dressing with champagne vinegar and light vegetable oil. Feel free to add any other herbs you wish to this light slaw. It goes well as a topping to fish tacos or as a side to ribs or chicken.

4 cups nappa cabbage, shredded, chopped

2 cups fresh burnet leaves, loosely packed

3 sprigs fresh purple basil, chiffonade

20 fresh nasturtium leaves

5 fresh nasturtium flowers, petals removed

2 Tbsp. champagne or white wine vinegar

2 Tbsp. guava nectar

¼ cup vegetable oil

½ tsp. kosher salt

1. IN A LARGE BOWL, combine nappa cabbage and next four ingredients. In a small mason jar with a screw top lid, combine vinegar, nectar, vegetable oil, and salt. Shake dressing vigorously until thickened. Add to cabbage mixture. Toss to coat. Cover and refrigerate until ready to serve.

SERVINGS: 4 | SOURCE: Little Rusted Ladle

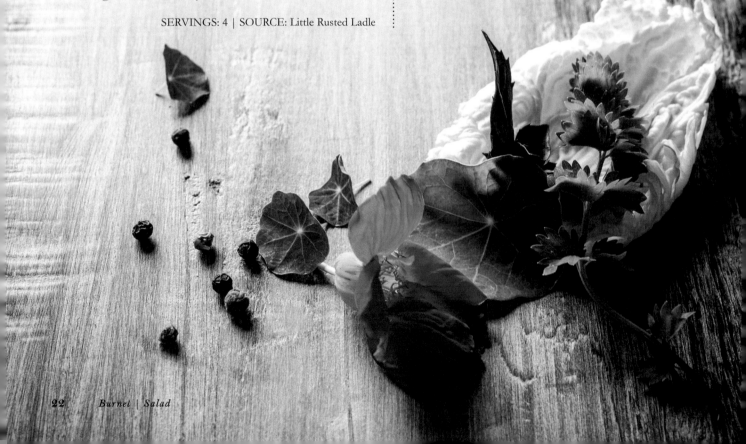

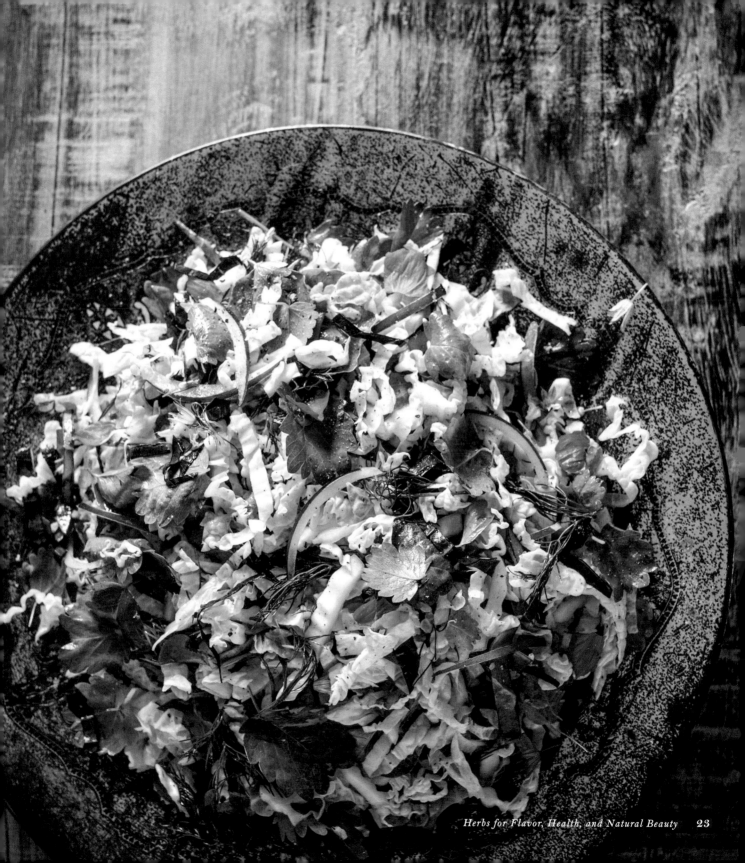

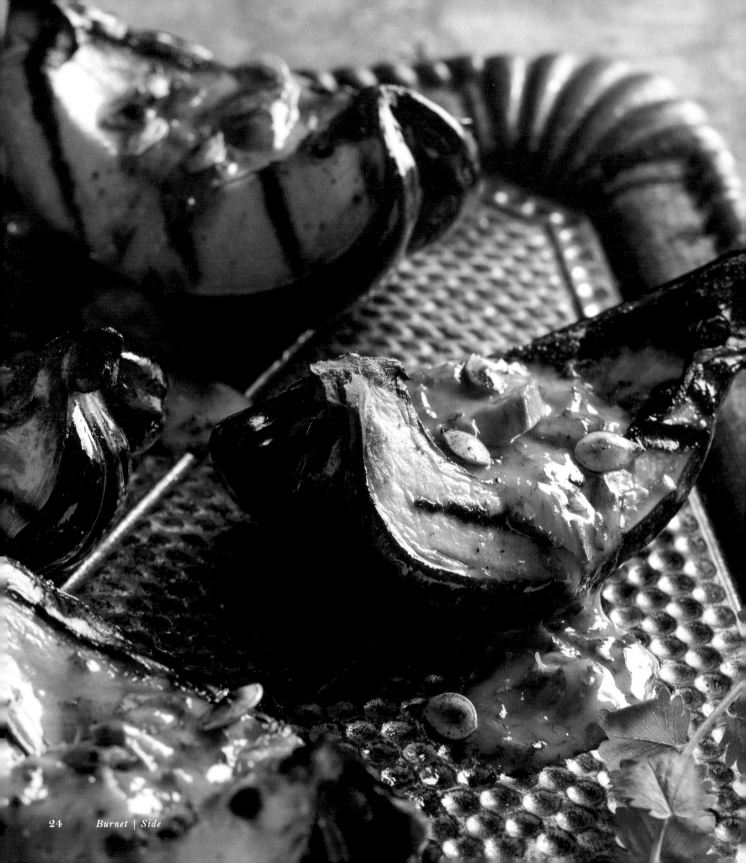

GRILLED ACORN SQUASH WITH RHUBARB BURNET BUTTER

Squash gets a dramatic flavor infusion with this unique herb butter. The tartness of the rhubarb combined with fresh herbs goes great with the slightly smoky flavor of the grilled squash.

1 Tbsp. light olive oil

1 whole acorn squash, quartered

¼ tsp. black pepper

1 tsp. kosher salt, divided

2 stalks fresh rhubarb, trimmed

¼ cup water

3 Tbsp. honey

1 stick unsalted butter, softened

2 Tbsp. burnet leaves, chopped

1 Tbsp. fresh pineapple sage leaves, chopped

2 tsp. fresh lemon thyme leaves

1. Preheat gas grill to medium heat. Drizzle olive oil over squash, then rub squash with your hands to completely coat squash. Season with pepper and half of the salt. Place squash flesh-side down directly over heat. Grill for 4–5 minutes until charred slightly, turning once halfway through. Place rhubarb stalks on grill across grates to prevent squash from falling into grill. Grill for 1–2 minutes or until softened and slightly charred. Transfer rhubarb to a plate and set aside.

2. Transfer squash quarters to a 2-quart casserole dish and add ¼ cup water to the pan. Cover with aluminum foil and bake at 350 degrees for 20 minutes or until cooked through. Keep warm. While squash is finishing in the oven, make butter.

3. FOR RHUBARB BURNET BUTTER, place grilled rhubarb and honey in a blender or food processor. Pulse about ten seconds or until smooth. Transfer mixture to a medium size bowl, then stir butter, herbs, and remaining salt into rhubarb with a rubber spatula. Serve rhubarb burnet butter over warm squash. Sprinkle additional burnet leaves over squash and serve.

SERVINGS: 4 | SOURCE: Little Rusted Ladle

CEDAR GRILLED SALMON WITH BURNET SAUCE

The aromatic scent of charred cedar combined with the fresh flavors of burnet and mint dressing creates an irresistible combination that will please the palate. For a gourmet presentation, serve salmon with grilled asparagus and forbidden rice. Garnish with fresh herbs if desired.

4 cedar planks

½ cup vegetable oil, divided

¼ cup soy sauce

1 Tbsp. honey

½ tsp. sesame oil

4 salmon filets

1 cup fresh burnet leaves

1 Tbsp. fresh mint, chopped

2 Tbsp. rice wine vinegar

4 garlic chives, chopped

1 tsp. curry powder

1 garlic clove, minced

1 tsp. chili paste

1. Place cedar planks in a 13 x 9 pan. Cover planks with water and weigh down with a bowl of water. Soak planks for 30 minutes.

2. FOR SALMON MARINADE, in a small bowl, combine ¼ cup vegetable oil, soy sauce, honey, and sesame oil. Whisk mixture with a fork. Pour marinade onto a dinner size plate. Place salmon filets flesh-side down over marinade. Let sit at room temperature for 30 minutes while grill preheats.

3. Preheat gas grill to medium heat (about 350 degrees). If using charcoal, place coals in the center of grill, cover with lighter fluid, and wait five minutes before lighting. Light coals and let burn until gray.

4. FOR BURNET SAUCE, combine ¼ cup of vegetable oil and remaining ingredients in a blender and process until smooth. Set aside while grilling salmon.

5. TO GRILL SALMON, remove cedar planks from water and let any excess water drip off. Place one salmon filet in the middle of each cedar plank. Place planks on hot grill, cover and cook for 10–15 minutes or until salmon is cooked through and cedar is slightly charred. Remove planks from grill and serve salmon topped with reserved burnet sauce.

SERVINGS: 4 | SOURCE: Little Rusted Ladle

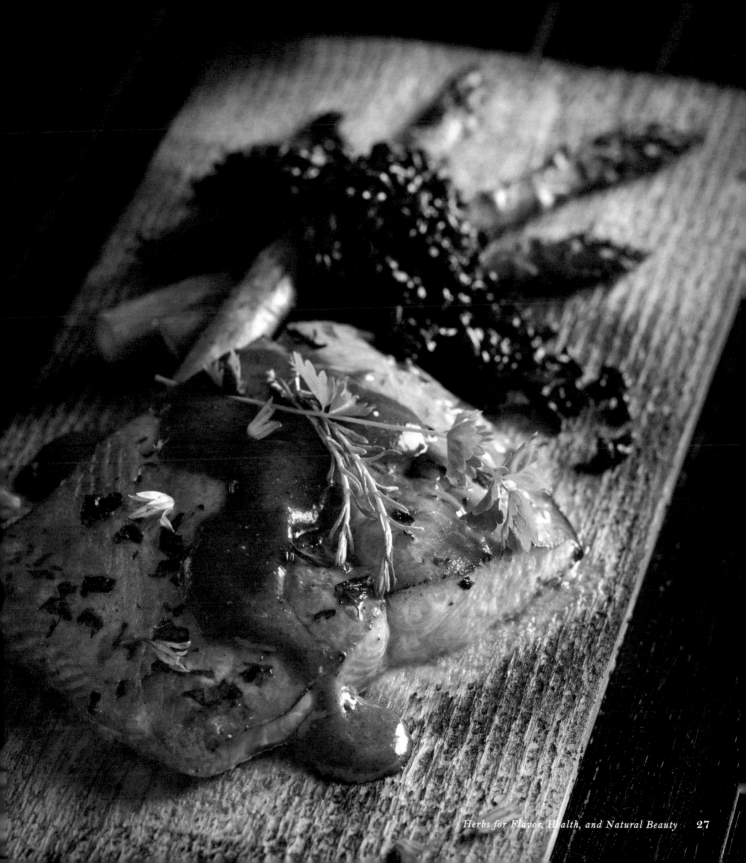

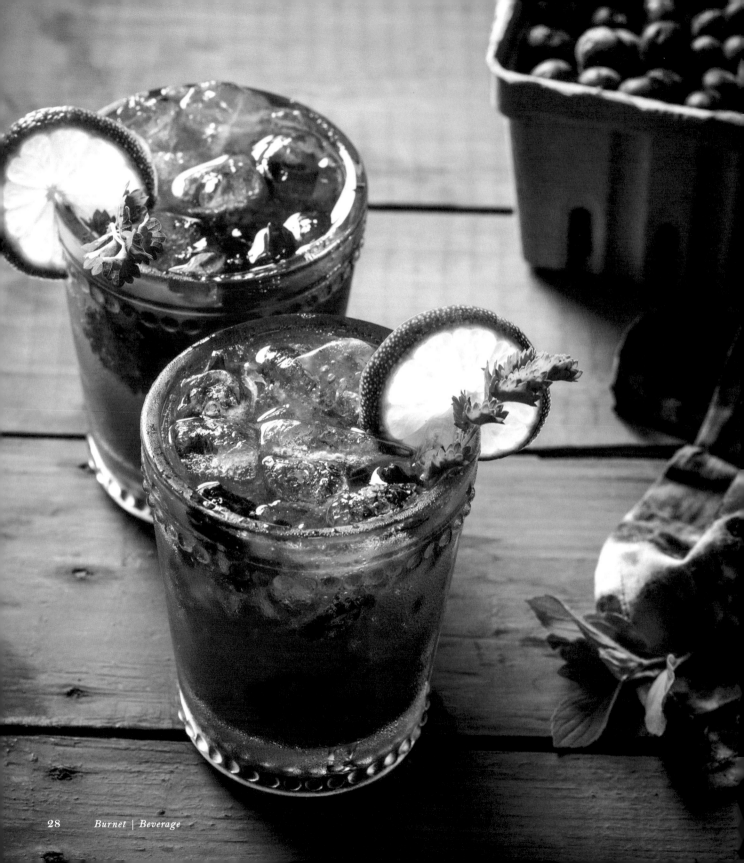

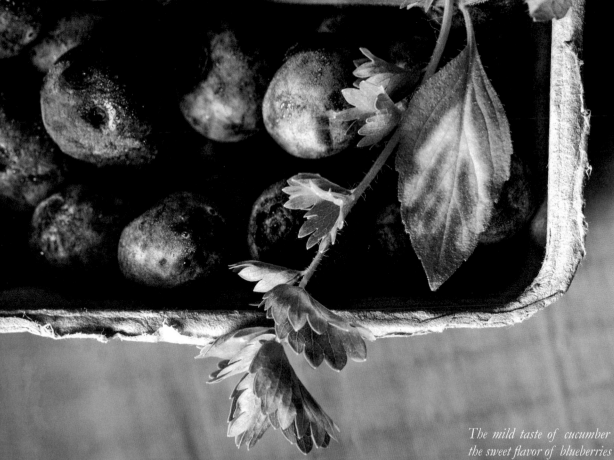

BLUEBERRY BURNET SPRITZER

1. IN A SMALL SAUCEPAN, simmer berries, sugar, and 1 cup of water over medium heat for 5–7 minutes or until blueberries have softened. Combine remaining tablespoon of water and cornstarch in a small dish and stir with a spoon until smooth. Stir into berry liquid. Simmer, stirring occasionally, until thickened, about two minutes. Transfer thickened berry mixture to a small container, cover, and refrigerate until cooled.

2. TO MAKE SPRITZERS, muddle a sprig each of burnet and mint leaves with a small wedge of lime in a rocks glass. Add ice, then 1½ oz. of lime soda. Spoon ¼ cup cooled berry mixture over ice. Top with ¼ of the non-alcoholic ginger beer and seltzer. Garnish with fresh burnet, mint, or lime and serve immediately.

SERVINGS: 4 | SOURCE: Little Rusted Ladle

The mild taste of cucumber combined with the sweet flavor of blueberries and fresh mint create a light and refreshing combination that's perfect on a hot summer day.

....

½ cup fresh blueberries

¼ cup fresh raspberries

⅓ cup sugar

½ cup water plus 1 Tbsp., divided

1 Tbsp. cornstarch

4 sprigs young burnet leaves

4 sprigs fresh mint

½ fresh lime, halved

Ice

6 oz. lemon lime soda

12 oz. non-alcoholic
ginger beer or ginger ale

1 cup seltzer

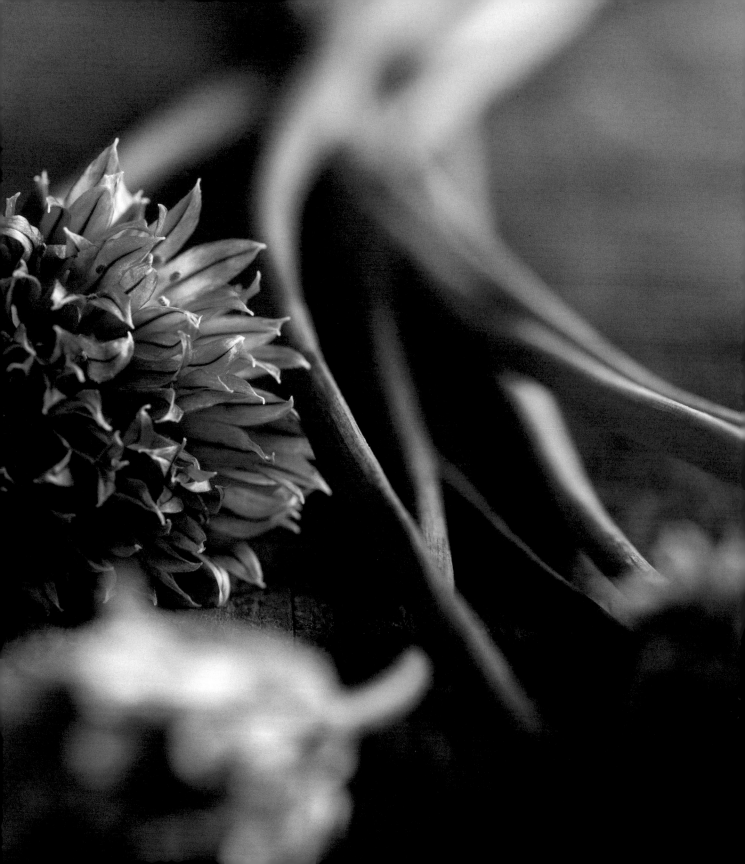

Chapter 3:
CHIVES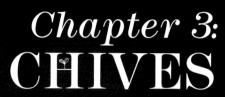

*T*his mild, long herb seems to be an offspring to the green onion. They may be similar in both genus and species, but they are not the same. In many ways, chives bring more to the table. For example, chives (both regular chives and garlic chive varieties) produce beautiful edible flowers in either the spring or late summer. Both are fabulous and are considered by many to be one of the best edible flowers produced by Mother Nature. Common chives produce a wonderful light purple flower that, with closer inspection, is actually a cluster of dozens of mini flowers each with its own stem. Garlic chives produce a delicate white flower. Pluck these little gems from the main bulb and sprinkle them on salads or fish or add them to dips or spreads. They also make a fabulous herb butter adding not only flavor, but color as well. When the chive blossoms bloom, cut them all down to the ground and you may be blessed with a second harvest in late summer. If not, no worries; unlike green onions, which are a one and done vegetable, you'll still get a healthy amount of the chive stems all summer, which will grow back almost as quickly as you cut them.

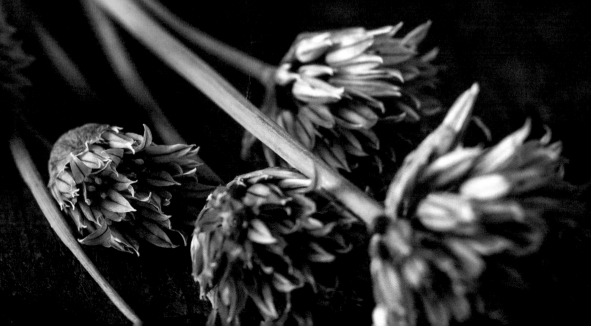

MINI CHIVE BLOSSOM CHEESE BALLS WITH CHIVE PICKS

These cute little cheese balls are a great way to use the blossoms of the chives. You can also use the stalks as picks. Use purple petals from regular chives in the spring and white ones from garlic chives in the summer. Feel free to substitute any semi-soft cheese you wish.

½ cup colby cheese, shredded

½ cup smoked gouda cheese, shredded

½ cup mascarpone or cream cheese, softened

2 Tbsp. unsalted butter, softened

1 tsp. spicy brown mustard

1 tsp. maple syrup

¼ tsp. black pepper

3 Tbsp. fresh chives, minced

1 Tbsp. fresh parsley, minced

1 tsp. fresh basil leaves, minced

1 tsp. lemon verbena leaves, minced

¼ cup slivered almonds, toasted, finely chopped

2 chive blossoms, purple or white, petals reserved

2 chive blossom stems, cut into 2-to 3-inch pieces

½ whole honeycrisp apple, cut into ¼ inch slices

1. FOR CHEESE BALLS, in a small mixing bowl, combine colby cheese and next 6 ingredients. Blend with a hand mixer on medium speed until smooth. Form cheese mixture by heaping tablespoons into balls. Place balls on a sheet pan lined with wax paper. Refrigerate for one hour or until firm. Meanwhile, make herb coating.

2. IN A SMALL BOWL, combine minced chives and next 5 ingredients. Stir to combine. Place cheese balls in herb mixture one at a time, lightly pressing mixture into each ball. Return balls to sheet pan. Place chive picks in the top of each ball, cover and refrigerate for one hour. Serve cheese balls on apple slices and enjoy.

SERVINGS: 6 | SOURCE: Little Rusted Ladle

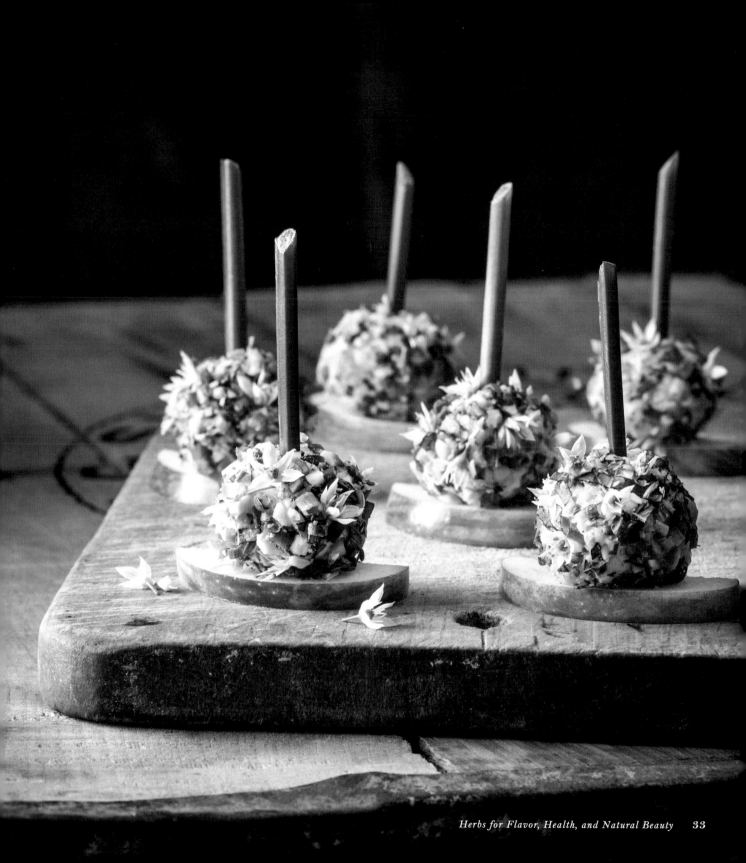

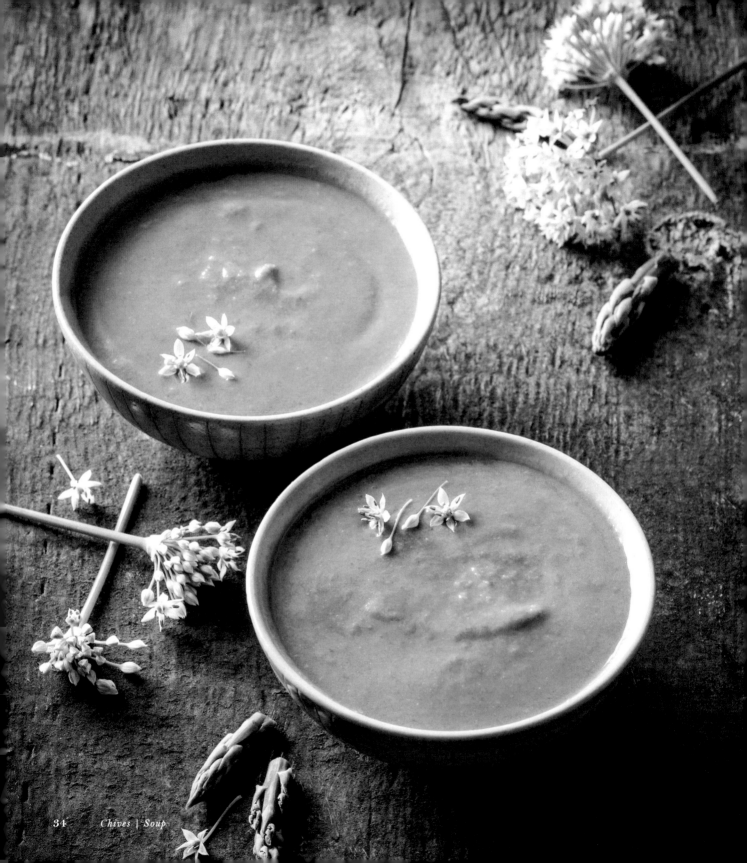

GARLIC CHIVE & ASPARAGUS SOUP WITH CHIVE BLOSSOMS

This healthy soup is best in the spring when purple chive blossoms and asparagus are at their peak freshness. Adding garlic chives adds a subtle garlic flavor, and making this soup in late summer gives you the option of using the beautiful garlic chive blossoms, which are white.

1. In a medium saucepan over medium heat, combine vegetable broth and next four ingredients. Bring to a simmer, then add asparagus. Cook until crisp-tender, about seven minutes. Add spinach and simmer an additional 2–3 minutes.

2. Transfer mixture along with fresh chives and avocado pieces to a blender or food processor. Puree until smooth. Season with salt and pepper. Pour into bowls and serve topped with garlic or regular chive blossom flowers.

SERVINGS: 4 | SOURCE: Little Rusted Ladle

1 cup vegetable broth

1 cup coconut water

½ cup almond milk, unsweetened

¼ cup soy sauce

2 garlic cloves, minced

8 stalks fresh asparagus, trimmed, cut into 1-inch pieces

1 cup baby spinach, washed

1½ cups fresh chives, chopped

1 avocado, skin removed, cut into pieces

4 garlic (or regular) chive blossoms, optional

Salt and pepper to taste

BRUSSEL SPROUT LEAF SALAD WITH CHIVE BLOSSOM VINAIGRETTE

This salad is the meeting of two seasons. Winter passing the torch on to spring. Baby cabbage with a light onion flavor and the added crunch of granola with fresh, sweet orange. Hello, spring. Use the chive blossom vinaigrette in place of any mild vinegar for dressings, marinades, or pickled vegetables.

1 Tbsp. chive blossoms or white wine vinegar, see step 1 below for recipe

2 tsp. honey

4 garlic chives, chopped

2 tsp. chive blossom petals

2 Tbsp. vegetable oil

¼ tsp. salt and pepper to taste

1 Tbsp. coconut oil

4 cups brussel sprout leaves

2 Tbsp. granola, prepared

1 navel orange, peeled, cut into segments

1. FOR CHIVE BLOSSOM VINEGAR, place 1 cup washed and dried chive blossoms in a clean canning jar. Pour 1 cup warm vinegar over chives. Cover with lid and store in a cool, dark place for four days to one month. Use as desired for dressings or marinades.

2. FOR CHIVE BLOSSOM VINAIGRETTE, in a small bowl, combine prepared chive blossom vinegar, honey, garlic chives and chive blossom petals. Slowly whisk in olive oil until thickened. Season to taste with salt and pepper. Set aside.

3. FOR BRUSSEL SPROUTS, preheat a large skillet over medium heat. Add coconut oil, then add brussel sprout leaves and granola. Quickly sauté leaves until bright green and lightly wilted, but still crisp, 2–3 minutes. Remove from heat. Add reserved dressing and toss to coat. Season with salt and pepper. Transfer warm salad to a serving dish or individual plates. Add orange segments and additional chive blossom flowers if desired. Serve.

SERVINGS: 4 | SOURCE: Little Rusted Ladle

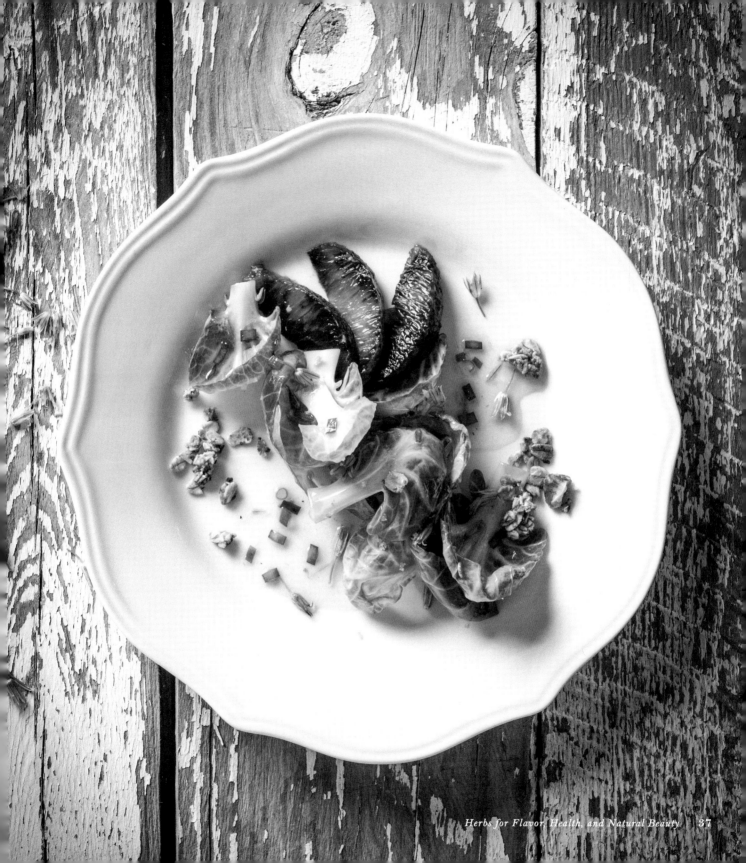

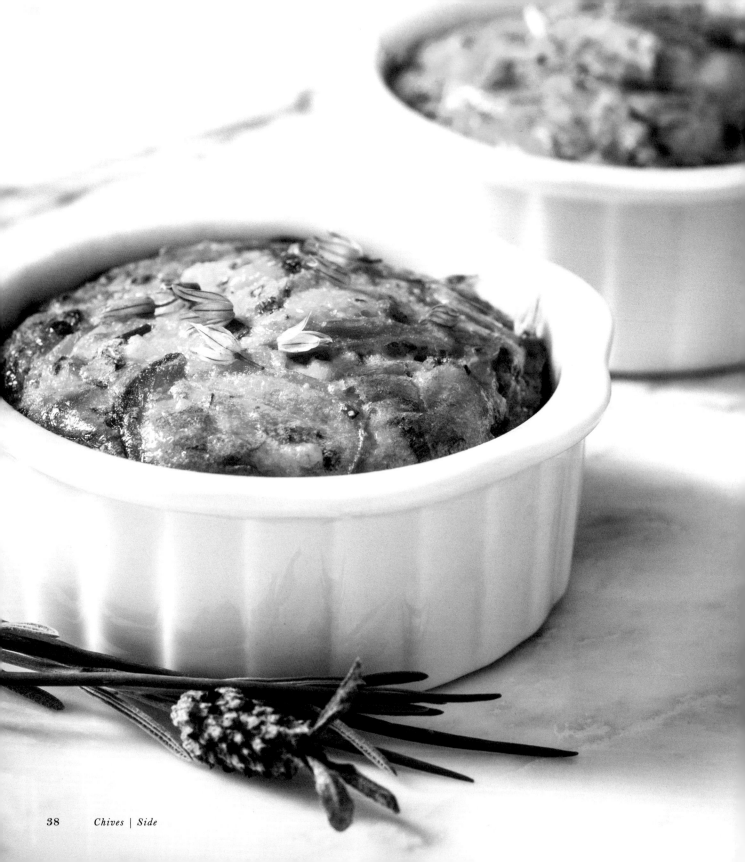

VIDALIA ONION AND CHIVE SOUFFLÉ

Spring is a wonderful time of year. It means the start of fresh, local vegetables and herbs. One of these treats is sweet vidalia onions. The sugars really come out of these when they are slow cooked. Add the mild flavor of fresh chives, some swiss cheese, and farm fresh eggs, and you've got a great side dish that goes great with meats. Or add chicken or more veggies, and serve them on their own.

1 Tbsp. light olive oil

1 Tbsp. unsalted butter

2 medium vidalia or sweet yellow onions, peeled and thinly sliced (about 3 cups)

4 large eggs, beaten

⅓ cup self-rising white cornmeal mix

1 cup whole milk

½ cup shredded baby swiss cheese

¼ cup chopped fresh chives

1 tsp. kosher salt

1 tsp. fresh lavendar flowers, optional

½ tsp. fresh ground black pepper

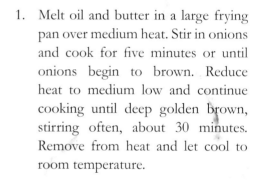

1. Melt oil and butter in a large frying pan over medium heat. Stir in onions and cook for five minutes or until onions begin to brown. Reduce heat to medium low and continue cooking until deep golden brown, stirring often, about 30 minutes. Remove from heat and let cool to room temperature.

2. While onions are cooling, preheat oven to 375 degrees. Spray four 8–12 oz. ramekins with nonstick spray. Combine eggs with remaining ingredients in a medium size bowl.

3. Pour egg mixture evenly into ramekins. Place on a baking sheet and bake for 25 minutes or until soufflés are well-risen, golden brown, and egg is completely cooked. Remove from oven and serve immediately.

SERVINGS: 4 | SOURCE: Little Rusted Ladle

FRESH CHIVE POPOVERS

This classic egg dish often referred to as "yorkshire pudding" gets an upgrade with the addition of fresh herbs including chives, parsley, and rosemary. The mild onion flavor really stands out. For even more chive flavor, add some chive blossom butter (see Grilled Shrimp with Chive Blossom Butter on page 43 for the recipe).

¾ cup milk

2 large eggs, beaten

½ cup unbleached flour

¼ cup dry roasted macadamia nuts, finely ground

2 Tbsp. chopped fresh chives

2 tsp. chopped fresh parsley

2 tsp. chopped fresh rosemary leaves

2 Tbsp. chive blossom or unsalted butter, melted

¼ tsp. salt

Fresh chopped chives for garnish, optional

1. Whisk all ingredients together in a medium size bowl. Cover bowl and refrigerate while oven preheats.

2. Preheat oven to 450 degrees. Place popover pan or six 8 oz. custard cups on a large sheet pan. Spray with nonstick spray. Fill each one $^2/_3$ full. Bake on a lower rack for 15 minutes without opening oven. Reduce heat to 350 degrees and bake an additional 20–25 minutes or until well-risen and golden brown. Remove from oven, pierce tops with a knife, and serve immediately with extra chive blossoms or unsalted butter and sprinkle with additional chopped chives if desired.

SERVINGS: 4 | SOURCE: Little Rusted Ladle

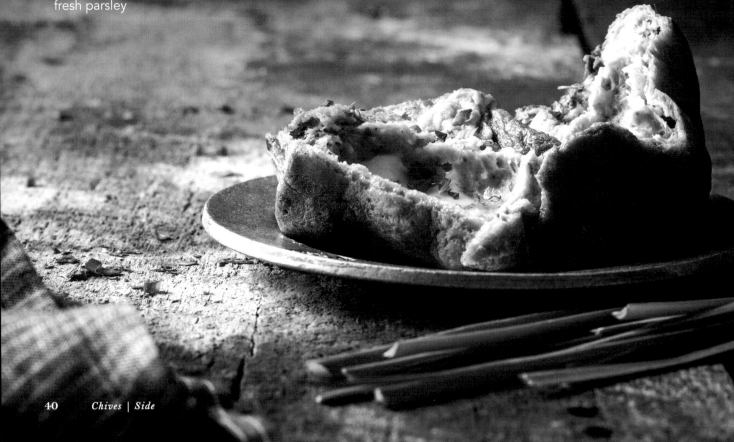

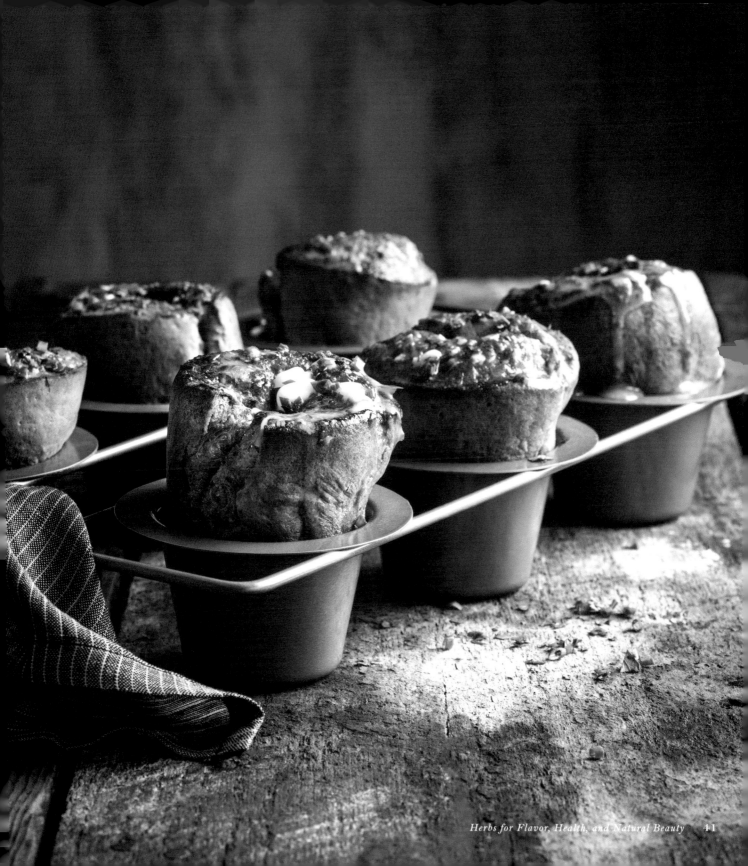

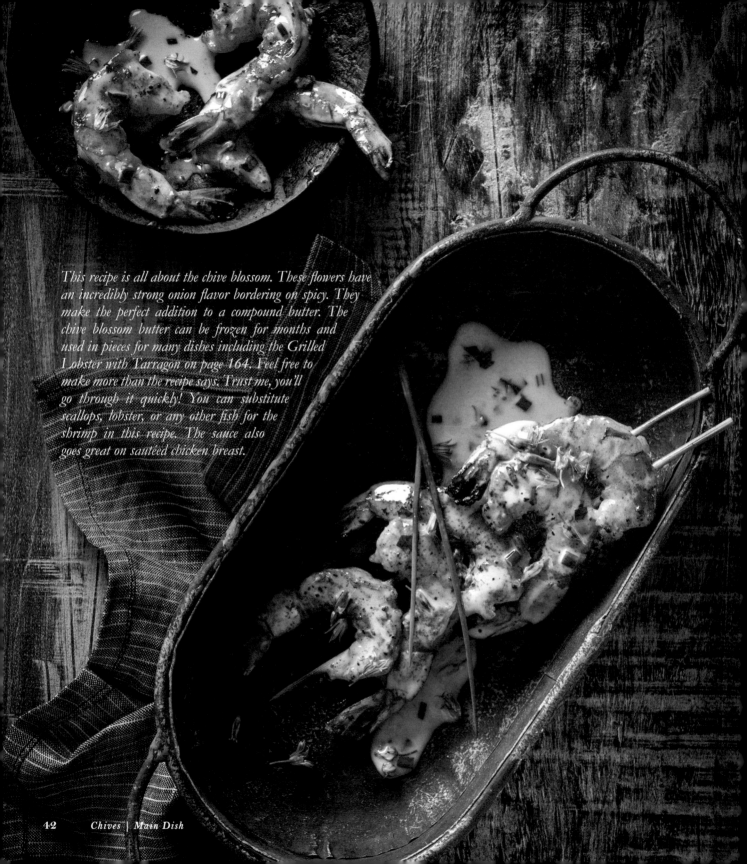

This recipe is all about the chive blossom. These flowers have an incredibly strong onion flavor bordering on spicy. They make the perfect addition to a compound butter. The chive blossom butter can be frozen for months and used in pieces for many dishes including the Grilled Lobster with Tarragon on page 164. Feel free to make more than the recipe says. Trust me, you'll go through it quickly! You can substitute scallops, lobster, or any other fish for the shrimp in this recipe. The sauce also goes great on sautéed chicken breast.

GRILLED SHRIMP WITH CHIVE BLOSSOM BUTTER

1 lb. unsalted butter, softened

8 ea. chive blossoms (purple), stems removed

8 ea. chives, chopped

2 Tbsp. fresh parsley, finely chopped

1 tsp. kosher salt

2 cloves Garlic, minced

1 Tbsp. Fresh lemon juice

2 tsp. Dijon mustard, optional

1½ lbs. large shrimp (16–20 count), peeled and deveined (tail on)

½ cup reduced sodium chicken broth, such as reisling

½ cup heavy cream, warmed

Fresh chive blossoms for garnish, optional

1. FOR THE CHIVE BLOSSOM BUTTER, beat butter and next seven ingredients with a hand mixer on low speed until well blended. Transfer mixture to a 1-gallon re-sealable plastic bag. Remove as much air as possible, seal, then cut the tip off one end of the bag, leaving about a 1½-inch opening. Position a sheet of parchment paper 12 X 6 in. on a flat surface. Pipe butter lengthwise along the long edge of the parchment paper 1" from the edge. Carefully roll the paper over the butter. Gently even the butter until you have an even roll of wrapped butter. Place on a sheet pan and freeze until hard (about 1 hour). Unroll butter and place on a cutting board. Cut into 1-inch pieces. Transfer pieces to a container or freezer bag and freeze until needed.

2. FOR GRILLED SHRIMP, saodk skewers in water for one hour. Preheat barbecue grill. Thread 4–5 shrimp onto each skewer. In a small bowl, melt two pieces of prepared chive blossom butter.

3. Brush skewers of shrimp with melted butter. Grill over direct heat for 2–3 minutes per side or until opaque and firm. Transfer to a plate and tent with foil. Keep warm while making sauce.

4. FOR SAUCE, in a small skillet, sauté garlic in 1 Tbsp. of chive blossom butter over medium heat until lightly browned. Add chicken broth and cook until broth is reduced to a glaze. Add cream and bring to a boil. Cook until reduced by half. Remove from heat and stir in 2 Tbsp. of chive blossom butter one at a time until melted, stirring continually. Season with salt and pepper. Serve over prepared shrimp skewers. Garnish with chive blossom flowers. Enjoy.

SERVINGS: 4 | SOURCE: Little Rusted Ladle

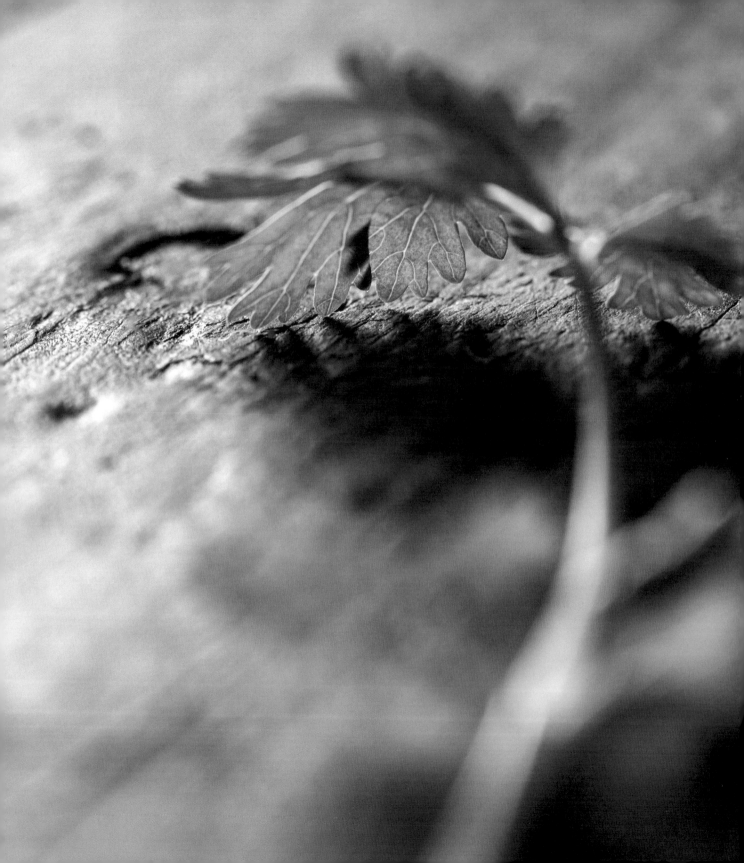

Chapter 4: CILANTRO

Cilantro could be one of the most used and versatile herbs on the planet. It has been used for over 3,500 years and can be found in many cultures and countries including Asia, Mexico, Europe, and Africa. Its uses are not limited to its fresh form, however. The dried seeds of cilantro are known as the flavorful spice coriander. It has medicinal uses as well, including being used as a diuretic to help remove heavy metals from the body and even to aid in joint problems when used externally. The next time you eat some salsa, or thai food, enjoy the flavor and look at that cilantro with new respect and admiration.

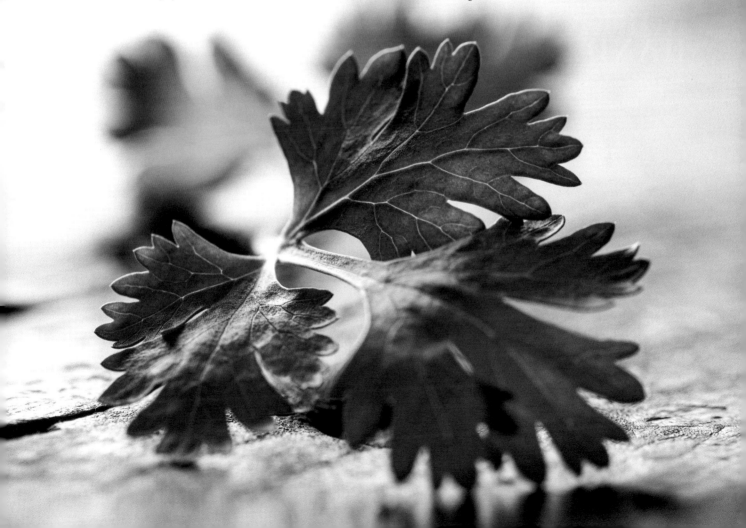

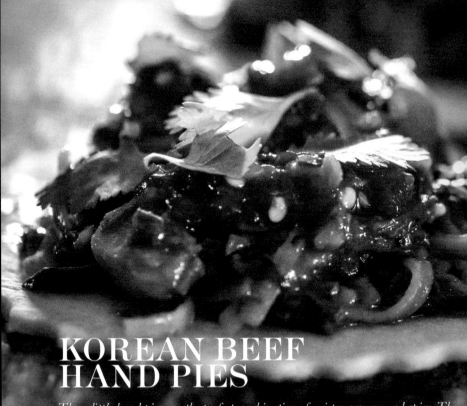

KOREAN BEEF HAND PIES

These little hand pies are the perfect combination of crispy, savory, and spicy. The cilantro may seem like a secondary ingredient, but without it, the flavor of these hand pies suffers. Pair these tasty treats with thai noodles or Jicama Salad and you have a filling meal. To serve as an entrée, spoon the mixture into a pie plate lined with one pie dough round. Top with cilantro, then top with remaining pie dough round. Top with sesame seeds and bake for one hour or until golden brown.

1 lb. boneless beef short ribs

½ cup chicken broth

¼ cup soy sauce

2 Tbsp. hoisin sauce

1 Tbsp. chili paste

1 Tbsp. thinly sliced green onion

1 tsp. ginger paste or grated ginger

1 tsp. minced garlic cloves

2 fresh shiitake mushrooms, stems removed, finely chopped

½ cup rice noodles

¼ cup fresh pea pods, cut into small pieces

2 refrigerated 9-inch pie dough rounds

1½ Tbsp. chili paste

½ cup fresh cilantro leaves, loosely packed

1 large egg, beaten

1 Tbsp. sesame seeds, flavored or plain

1. FOR FILLING, place short ribs in a 1½ quart slow cooker. In a medium size bowl, combine chicken broth and next seven ingredients. Pour mixture over short ribs. Move ribs around to coat with sauce. Cover slow cooker and turn power level to low. Cook for 5–6 hours or until meat is tender. Transfer meat to a bowl and let cool for 15–20 minutes. Meanwhile, skim fat from cooking liquid. Break noodles into 2-inch pieces and add to cooking liquid with pea pods. Shred meat with two forks. Add meat to noodle and pea pod mixture. Toss gently to combine. Cover and refrigerate filling until ready to assemble.

2. TO MAKE PIES, cut out eight 4-inch rounds using a can, cutter, or a small tart pan. Place rounds on a parchment-lined sheet pan. Spoon about ½ cup of beef mixture over eight dough rounds, leaving about ½-inch border. Preheat oven to 400 degrees. Spoon about a teaspoon of chili sauce over beef, then top with a Tbsp. of fresh cilantro leaves. Brush edges with beaten egg. Place remaining dough rounds over filling and carefully press edges together to seal. Brush tops with egg, then quickly sprinkle with sesame seeds. Bake for 20–25 minutes or until golden brown. Serve immediately. Enjoy.

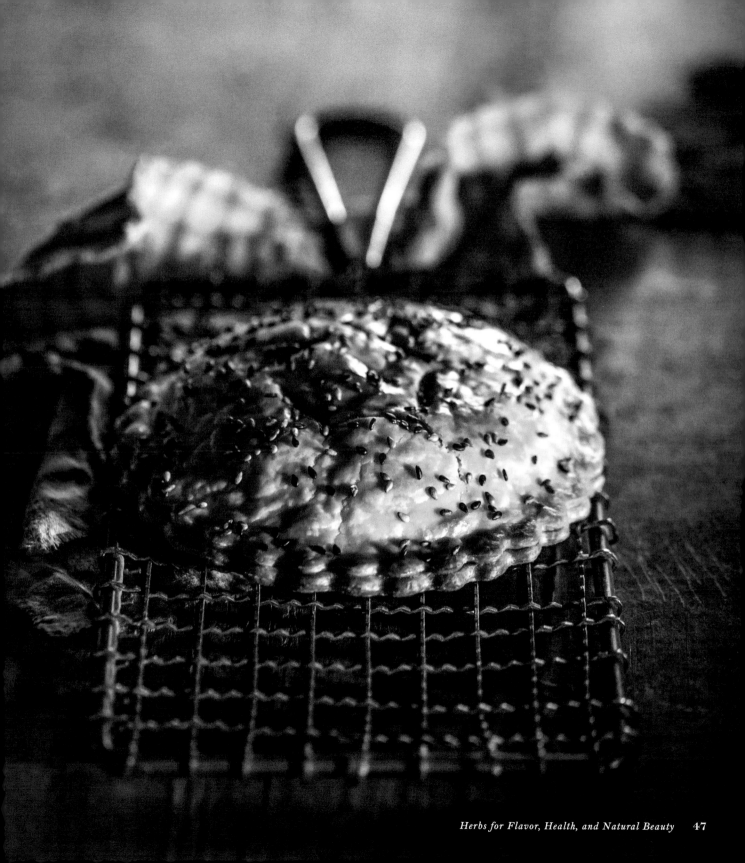

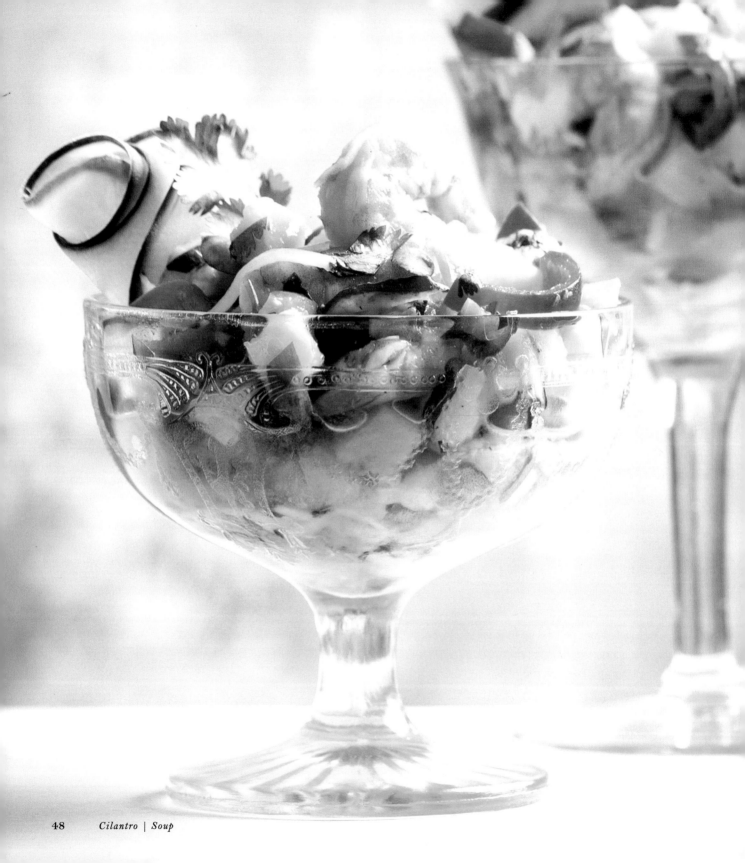

MANGO & SHRIMP CEVICHE

Fresh champagne mangos when in season are as sweet as honey. They are the perfect addition to this ceviche, and the cilantro does exactly what cilantro is supposed to do, make things taste better. You can make a mango salsa by eliminating the shrimp and all but one tablespoon of lime juice. Serve as is or with chicken, pork, or seafood.

½ lb. medium shrimp,
peeled, deveined, and halved

½ cup fresh lime juice, about 4 limes

½ cup diced fresh champagne mango

1 fresh habanero pepper, seeded, chopped

2 green onions, thinly sliced

½ shredded or thinly sliced cup radish

½ cup peeled and small diced Jicama

½ cup diced roma tomato

¼ cup diced red bell pepper

2 Tbsp. chopped fresh cilantro

1 Tbsp. extra virgin olive oil

1. Combine shrimp and lime juice in a medium glass bowl. Toss well to coat. Cover and refrigerate for 45 minutes. Fold in remaining ingredients. Cover and refrigerate for one hour or until shrimp is opaque in color. Serve as is or with tortilla chips or grilled baguette slices.

SERVINGS: 4 | SOURCE: Little Rusted Ladle

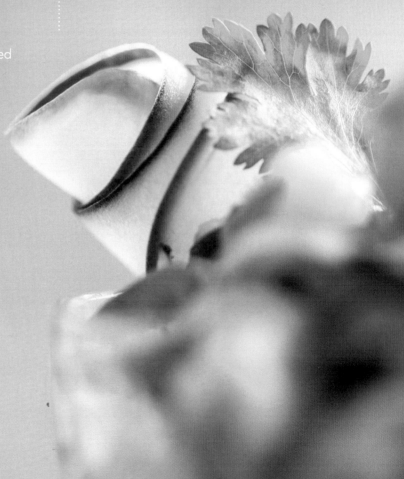

JICAMA AND PLUM SALAD WITH CILANTRO

This fresh salad highlights the beauty and flavor of fresh plums when they are in season. Try adding two or three different kinds for added color and flavor. Adding the cilantro serrano syrup adds a punch at the end, while the fresh cilantro leaves with help cool it down. If you don't want the heat of the serrano syrup, simply add another teaspoon of honey.

2½ cups peeled, cut into matchsticks jicama

3 plums, fresh, about 1½ cups, thinly sliced

½ cup loosely packed cilantro leaves

1 apricot, fresh, thinly sliced

2 tsp. honey

1 tsp. Sassy Cilantro Syrup, see Peach Slushies recipe, page 57, optional

1 Tbsp. extra virgin olive oil

¼ cup pumpkin seeds, roasted and salted

½ tsp. curry powder

1 tsp. coconut oil

1. FOR SALAD, in a large bowl, combine jicama and next three ingredients. Set aside

2. FOR DRESSING, in a small jar with a lid, combine honey, sassy cilantro syrup, and olive oil. Cover and shake vigorously until well-blended. Set aside.

3. FOR NUTS, in a small skillet over medium heat, combine pumpkin seeds, curry powder, and coconut oil. Sauté mixture for 2–3 minutes, stirring seeds often to keep from burning and until golden brown. Remove from heat and let cool.

4. Add dressing to bowl of jicama mixture and toss to coat. Transfer to a serving bowl and top with toasted pumpkin seeds. Serve.

SERVINGS: 4 | SOURCE: Little Rusted Ladle

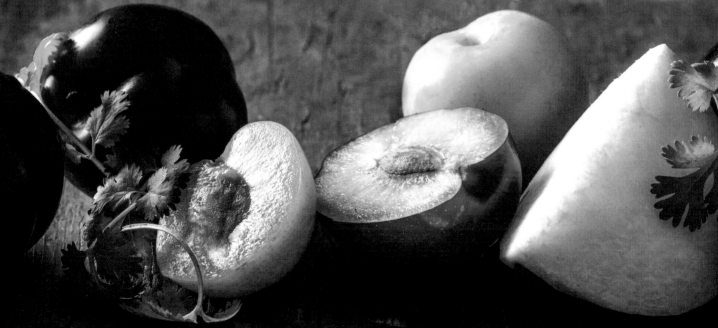

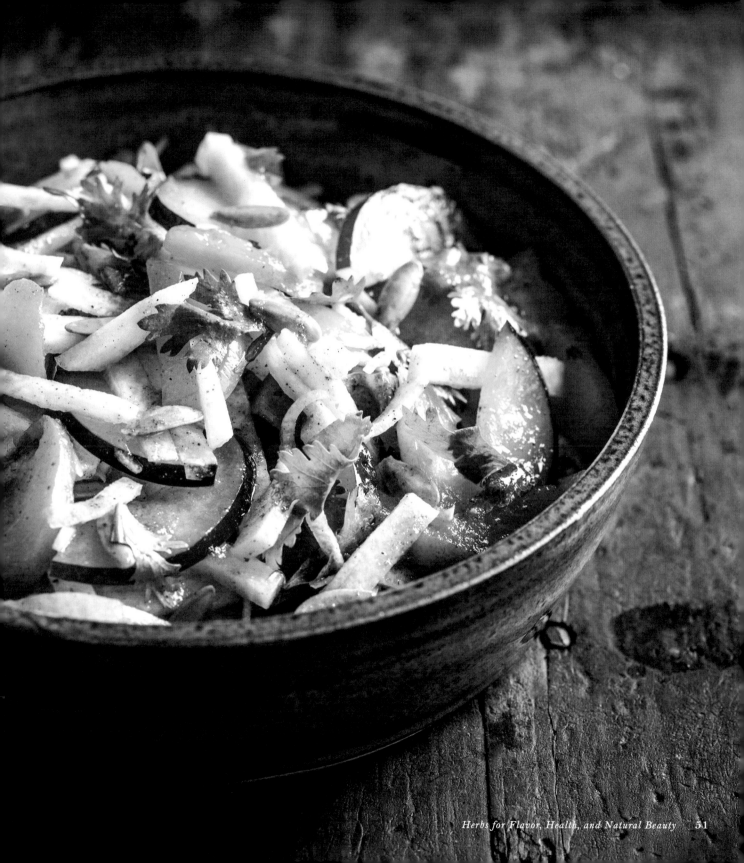

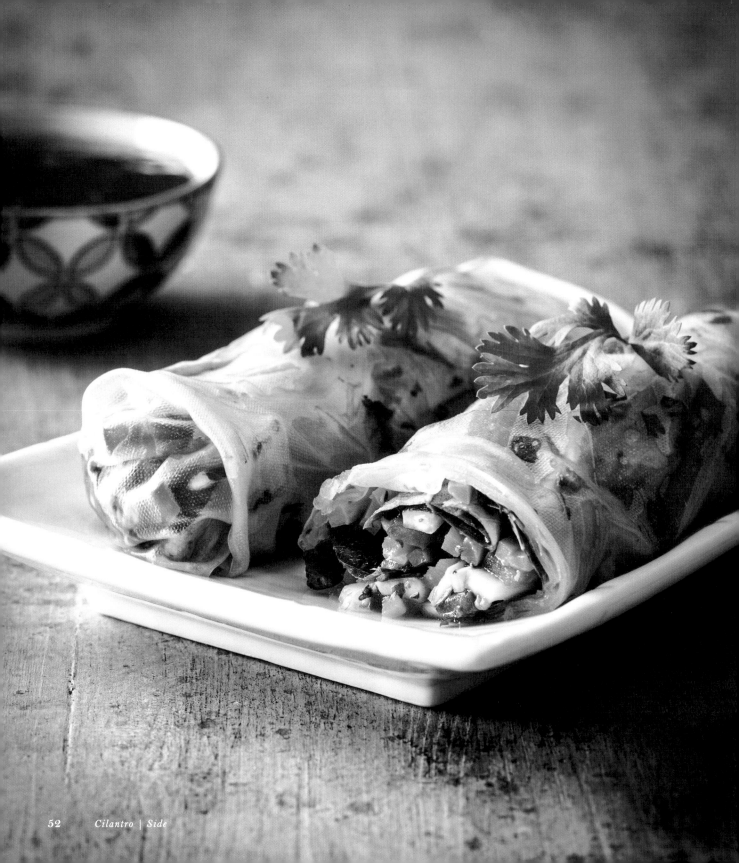

CILANTRO & VEGETABLE SPRING ROLLS

Spring rolls are a great way to wrap up all the fresh flavors of the garden in one neat, little, edible package. The flavor of fresh cilantro, basil, pineapple sage, mint, and lemon balm really jump off the taste buds. You can add chicken, shrimp, or rice noodles to the filling mix if you want to serve them more as a meal than a side dish.

1 cup fresh cilantro leaves, divided

2 Tbsp. peanut oil

1 Tbsp. fresh lime juice

½ tsp. kosher salt

1 tsp. sriracha chili sauce, optional

1 cup julienned red bell pepper

1 cup julienned yellow squash

1 cup julienned zucchini

1 cup shredded carrots

¼ cup chopped fresh chives

16 pineapple sage leaves

16 fresh basil leaves

16 lemon balm leaves

1 cup warm water

6 spring roll wrappers

6 oz. thai chili sauce, prepared, optional

1. Finely chop half of the cilantro and add to a small bowl with next 4 ingredients. Whisk until thickened slightly. Set aside while making spring rolls.

2. Combine red bell pepper, remaining cilantro, and next seven ingredients in a medium size bowl. Add reserved cilantro dressing and toss to coat.

3. TO ASSEMBLE SPRING ROLLS, pour warm water into a pie plate or deep plate. Dip one spring roll wrapper into warm water for about ten seconds or until slightly softened. Place wrapper flat on surface. Add a small bundle of vegetable mixture onto bottom third of wrapper. Fold bottom of wrapper over vegetables, then fold sides over towards the center. Roll spring roll over with the seam side down. Place on a platter or rectangular plate. Repeat with remaining spring roll wrappers and vegetables until all six spring rolls are made. If desired, serve with a side of thai chili sauce for dipping.

SERVINGS: 4 | SOURCE: Little Rusted Ladle

MOLE TURKEY TACOS WITH CILANTRO CREMA

The flavors of Oaxaca and Mexico City combine for this south-of-the-border favorite. A double dose of cilantro as both whole and a sauce adds wonderful flavor. Slow cooking the meat in a crockpot makes this dish a snap to prepare. You can substitute pork, chicken, or beef for the turkey if desired. To save time, prepared mole sauce can be purchased in most large grocery stores or mexican food markets.

20 oz. boneless turkey breast tenderloins	½ cup mexican crema or sour cream	12 taco size flour tortillas, 6-inch	¼ cup crumbled queso fresco,
8 oz. mole sauce, prepared	1 cup fresh cilantro leaves, divided	½ cup thinly sliced red onion	½ cup cherry tomatoes, quartered
½ cup chicken stock	Sprinkle of salt, optional	½ cup diced mango, 1 avocado, sliced	Hot sauce of choice, optional

1. FOR MOLE TURKEY, in a 1-quart crock-pot, combine turkey, mole sauce, and chicken stock. Cover and turn to low temperature. Cook for 4–5 hours or until turkey pulls easily with a fork. Transfer to a bowl and set aside to cool slightly, about 15 minutes. Shred mixture with two forks and fold in sauce until mixture is saucy. Transfer back to crock-pot and keep warm.

2. FOR CILANTRO CREMA, in a small blender or food processor, blend crema and half of cilantro until smooth and light green. Season with salt if desired. Set aside.

3. TO MAKE TACOS, grill tortillas over hot, open flame on grill or gas burner for 8–12 seconds or until slightly burnt in areas. Place on oven-proof plate, cover, and keep warm. Repeat with remaining tortillas. Place about ⅓ cup of hot mole turkey mixture in the center of one warmed tortilla. Top with 3–4 pieces each of red onion and mango. Add a slice of avocado, about a tablespoon of queso fresco, and a sprig of remaining fresh cilantro. Top with cilantro crema and hot sauce, if desired. Repeat with remaining tacos. Enjoy.

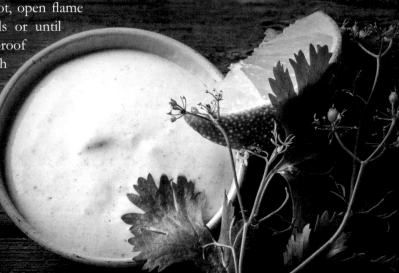

SERVINGS: 4 | SOURCE: Little Rusted Ladle

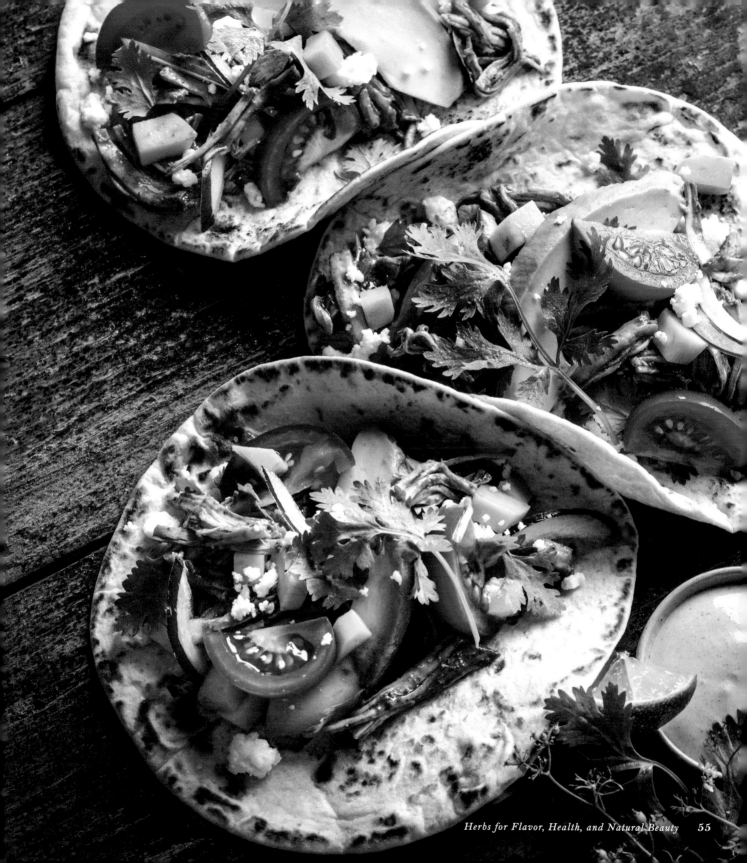

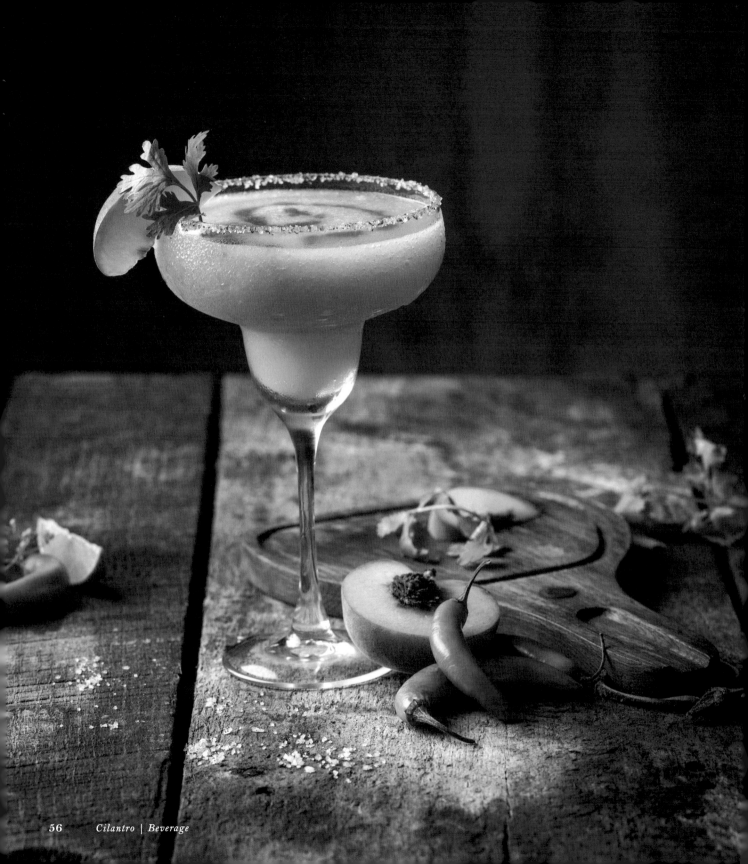

PEACH SLUSHIES WITH SASSY CILANTRO SYRUP

The taste of sweet peaches combined with the sweet and spicy cilantro syrup is a great way to enjoy summer.

....

2 serano chile peppers, stems removed

½ cup simple syrup

½ cup fresh cilantro leaves, loosely packed

4 cups frozen sliced peaches

6 oz. lemon lime soda

2 cups ice

2 Tbsp. fresh lime juice

1. FOR SASSY CILANTRO SYRUP, combine simple syrup and serano peppers in a small saucepan. Simmer on low for five minutes to release the oils in the peppers. Transfer to a blender and add cilantro. Blend until smooth. Store covered in a small container until needed.

2. FOR MARGARITA, combine peaches and remaining ingredients in a blender. Puree until smooth. Pour into salt-rimmed margarita glasses and serve with a spoonful of reserved sassy cilantro syrup swirled in. Enjoy.

SERVINGS: 4 | SOURCE: Little Rusted Ladle

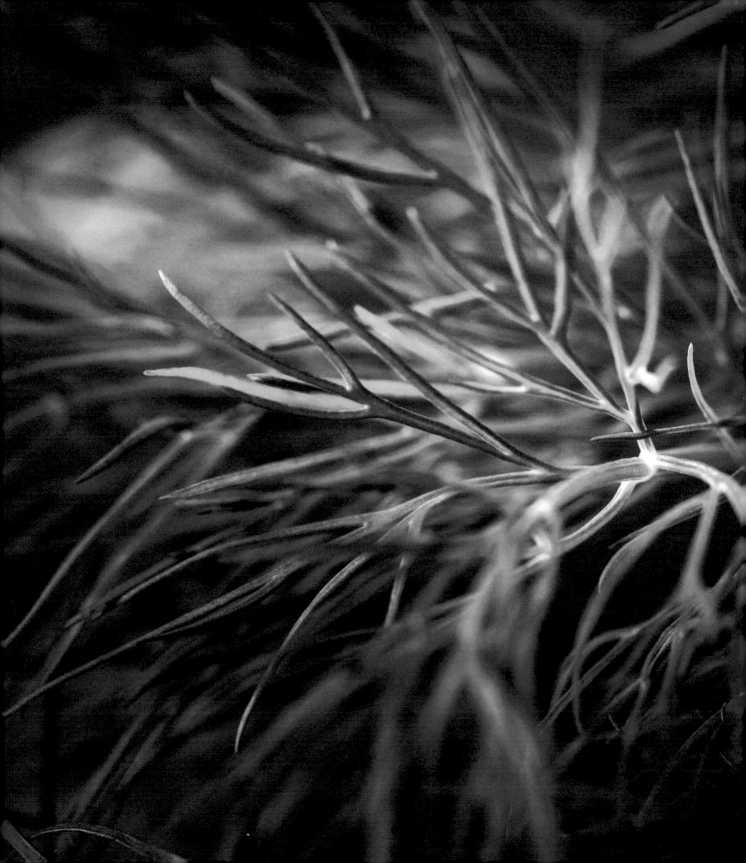

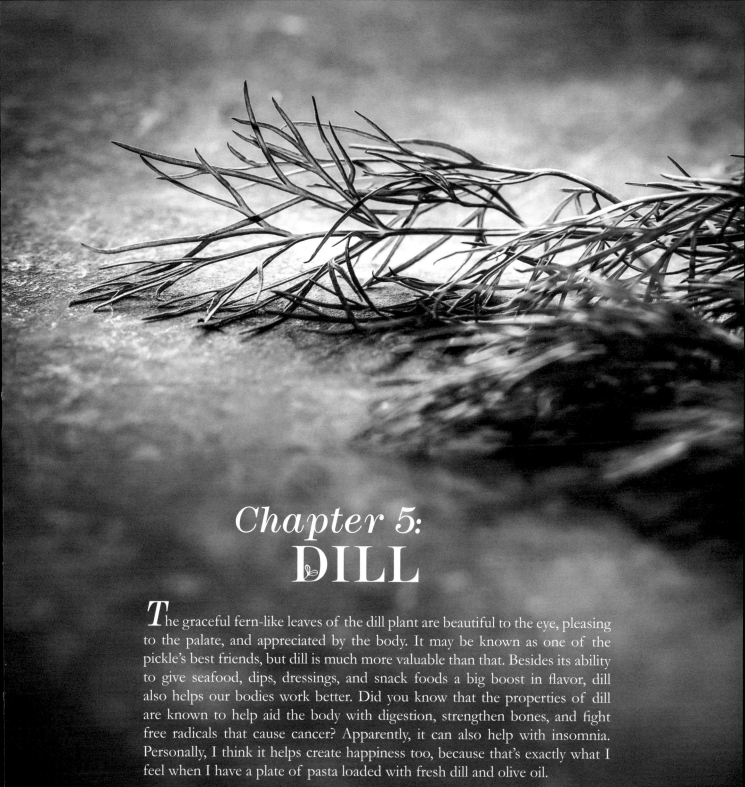

Chapter 5:
DILL

*T*he graceful fern-like leaves of the dill plant are beautiful to the eye, pleasing to the palate, and appreciated by the body. It may be known as one of the pickle's best friends, but dill is much more valuable than that. Besides its ability to give seafood, dips, dressings, and snack foods a big boost in flavor, dill also helps our bodies work better. Did you know that the properties of dill are known to help aid the body with digestion, strengthen bones, and fight free radicals that cause cancer? Apparently, it can also help with insomnia. Personally, I think it helps create happiness too, because that's exactly what I feel when I have a plate of pasta loaded with fresh dill and olive oil.

3-BEET & WATERCRESS TART WITH DILL

This recipe highlights the beauty and flavor of 4 different kinds of beets with three different kinds of cooking methods. The dill brings all the beet flavors together creating an earthy sweetness perfect for those late summer get-togethers. Chioggia beets are a beautifully sweet beet that has wonderful nutritional benefits. You can cook them prior to adding them to the tart if raw beets aren't your style.

1 sheet puff pastry, thawed

1 large egg white, beaten

2 tsps. sesame seeds

4 oz. goat cheese, softened

4 oz. cream cheese, softened

Salt and pepper to taste

2 Tbsp. chopped fresh dill

1 small chioggia beet, thinly sliced, optional

3 small pink beets, roasted, halved

4 small red beets, boiled until tender, peeled and sliced

2 small yellow beets, roasted, halved

½ cup watercress, washed

¼ cup microgreens, optional

1 Tbsp. pumpkin seeds, roasted, optional

1. FOR TART SHELL, preheat oven to 425 degrees. Unfold puff pastry onto a parchment-lined sheet pan. Cut ½ inch wide strips from all four sides of puff pastry and set aside. Brush remaining sheet of dough with egg white. Place reserved strips of puff pastry along edges on top of pastry sheet, creating a border. Press to seal. Brush edges of pastry with egg white. Using a fork, poke center area of puff pastry all over to prevent pastry from rising too much. Sprinkle sesame seeds along edges. Bake for 20–25 minutes or until golden brown. Remove from oven and let cool completely.

2. FOR CHEESE SPREAD, in a medium size bowl, combine goat cheese and cream cheese. Season to taste with salt and pepper.

3. TO ASSEMBLE PIZZA, spread cheese mixture over cooled puff pastry. Sprinkle dill over cheese mixture. Place beet slices, watercress, and microgreens evenly over cheese. Sprinkle with pumpkin seeds if desired. Cut into squares and serve.

SERVINGS: 6 | SOURCE: Little Rusted Ladle

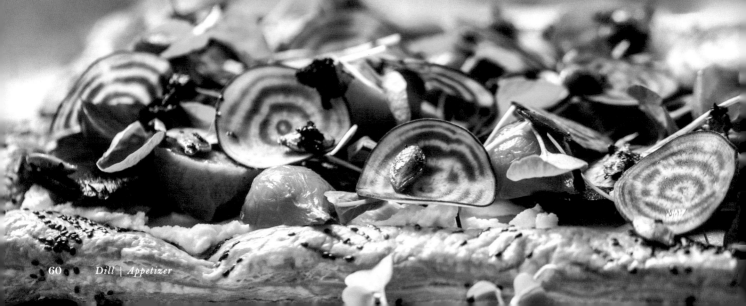

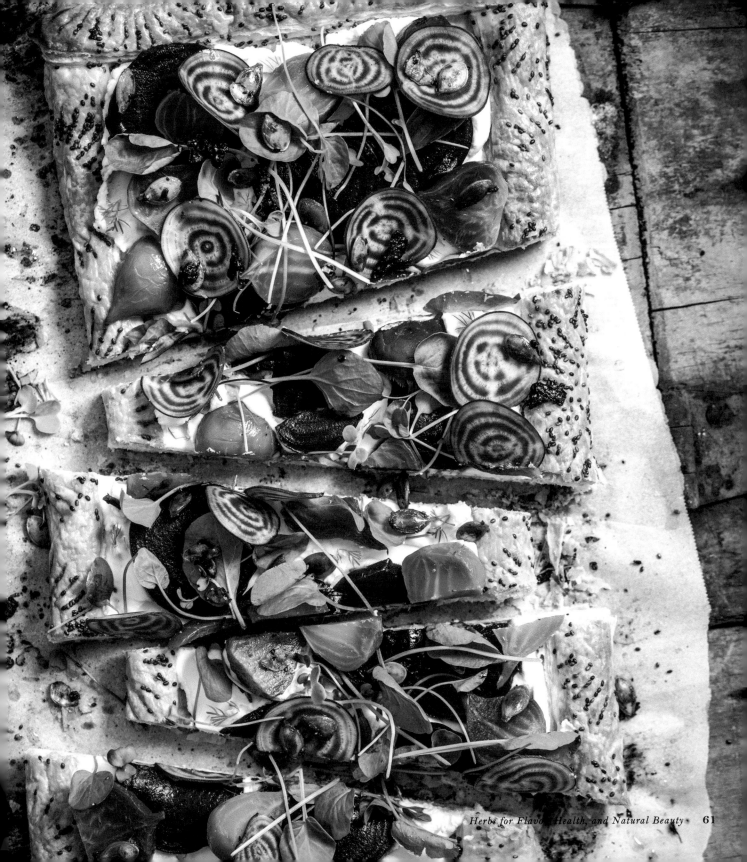

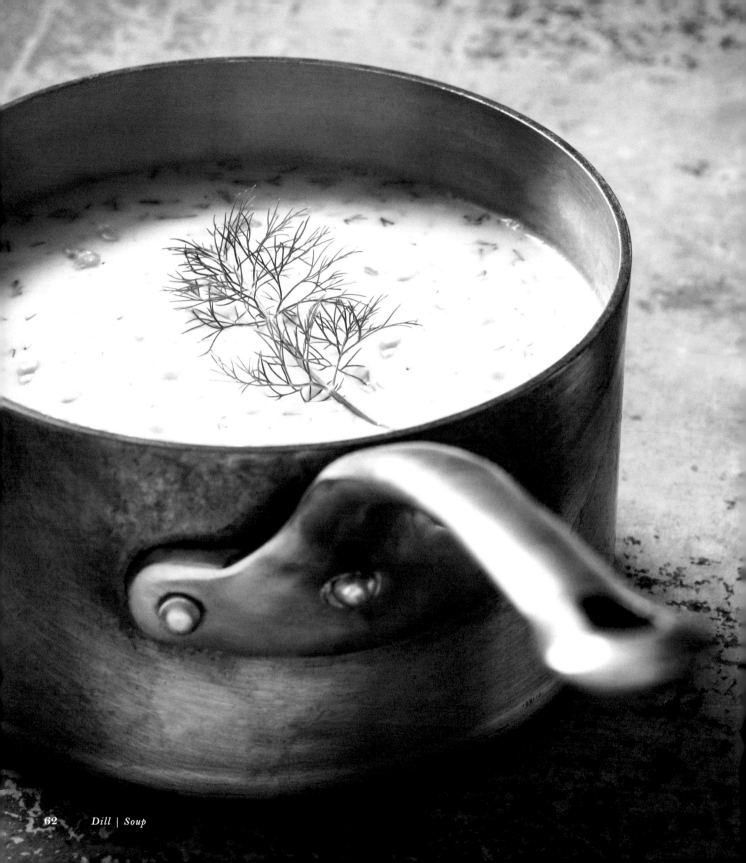

SWEET CORN & COCONUT SOUP WITH DILL

Sweet corn in the peak of season goes great with the flavors of coconut and dill. The cheese adds a little richness to the dish. By barely cooking the corn, the sweetness is maintained, giving the soup that fresh, sweet flavor found only during sweet corn season.

3 cups water

4 ears sweet corn, husks and silk removed

1½ Tbsp. cornstarch

1 (13.6 oz.) can coconut milk

1½ cups shredded smoked gouda cheese

½ cup chopped fresh dill

Salt and pepper to taste

1. IN A DUTCH OVEN OR LARGE SAUCEPAN, bring water to a simmer. Add corn. Cook for five minutes. Remove corn from water with a pair of tongs. Let corn cool enough to handle, then cut corn off of cobs and transfer kernels to a medium size bowl. Run the back of a knife over trimmed cobs to remove as much liquid as possible. Set pan of cooking water back on heat. Bring to a boil. Simmer for ten minutes or until liquid has reduced by one quarter. Remove any remaining silk from cooking liquid with a fine strainer.

2. Combine 2 tablespoons of cooking liquid with cornstarch in a small bowl. Whisk cornstarch mixture into hot cooking liquid. Bring to a boil, then reduce heat to simmer. Cook for two minutes. Whisk coconut milk and cheese into thickened cooking liquid. Simmer until cheese has melted into soup. Stir in reserved corn. Add dill, season to taste. Serve.

SERVINGS: 4 | SOURCE: Little Rusted Ladle

FRIED GREEN TOMATO NAPOLEAN

....

¼ cup cornstarch

1 large egg, beaten

½ cup gluten-free bread crumbs

3 Tbsp. fresh dill, divided

½ tsp. kosher salt

2 medium green tomatoes, sliced (8 slices)

4 strips bacon

Vegetable oil, optional

1 fresh peach, sliced (12–16 slices)

8 oz. burrata or fresh mozzarella cheese, sliced (8 slices)

20 cuban oregano leaves, washed

Fresh ground black pepper to taste

1. Put cornstarch, egg, and bread crumbs into three separate pie plates or paper plates. Add 2 tablespoons dill and salt to bread crumbs and stir to combine.

2. FOR TOMATOES, place one slice of tomato in cornstarch and coat both sides. Shake off excess. Dip slice into egg, then into bread crumbs, pressing breadcrumbs into both sides. Transfer tomato slice onto a foil-lined sheet pan and repeat process with remaining tomato slices. Set aside.

3. Fry bacon pieces in a large, heavy frying pan over medium heat until golden brown. Using a slotted spoon, transfer bacon to a plate lined with paper towels. Cut bacon into 1-inch pieces.

4. Fry 4–6 breaded tomato slices in rendered bacon grease on both sides until golden brown, about three minutes per side. Transfer fried tomatoes back to sheet pan and keep warm. Repeat with remaining tomato slices. Add some vegetable oil to pan during process if needed.

5. TO SERVE, place one tomato slice each on four plates. Top each slice with 2–3 slices of peach and one slice of burrata or fresh mozzarella cheese. Place another tomato slice on top and one more slice of burrata. Top with 2 more slices of peach. Finish with cuban oregano leaves, bacon pieces, and fresh ground black pepper. Serve immediately.

SERVINGS: 4 | SOURCE: Little Rusted Ladle

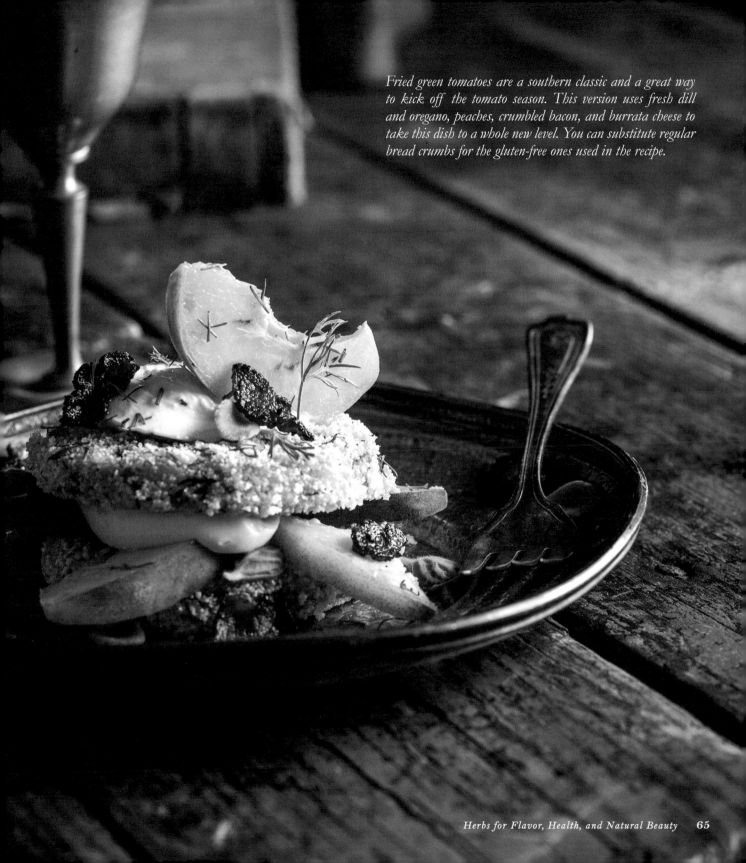

Fried green tomatoes are a southern classic and a great way to kick off the tomato season. This version uses fresh dill and oregano, peaches, crumbled bacon, and burrata cheese to take this dish to a whole new level. You can substitute regular bread crumbs for the gluten-free ones used in the recipe.

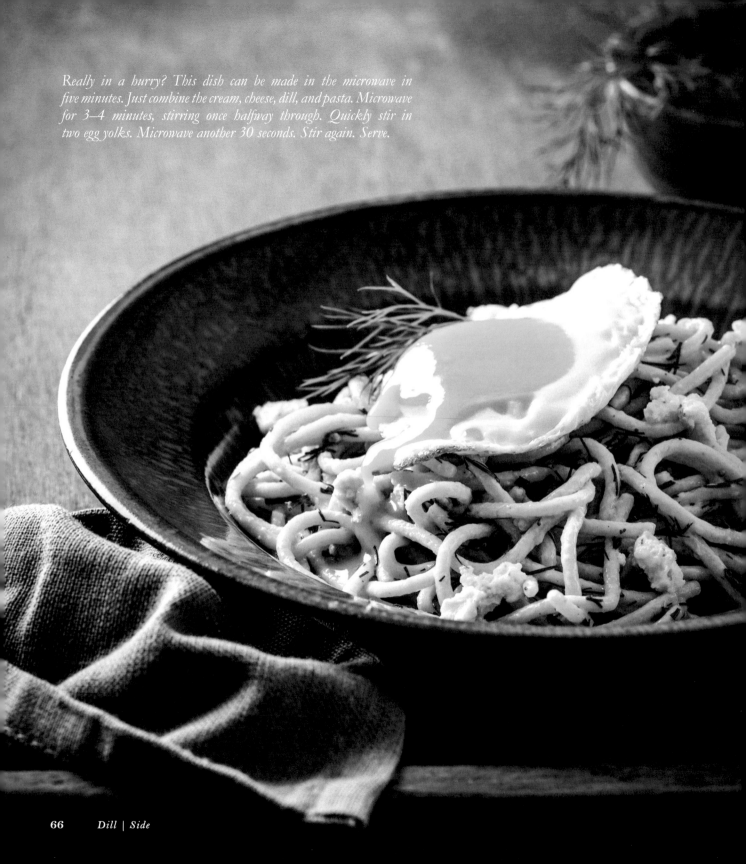

Really in a hurry? This dish can be made in the microwave in five minutes. Just combine the cream, cheese, dill, and pasta. Microwave for 3–4 minutes, stirring once halfway through. Quickly stir in two egg yolks. Microwave another 30 seconds. Stir again. Serve.

DILLED PASTA CARBONARA

Dill is one of those herbs that can be quickly added to a recipe, taking it to a different level. This playful variation to a classic carbonara without the pork is one of those recipes. It is a great way to use precooked pasta. The creamy boursin cheese, which is a garlic-and-herb-flavored soft cheese, can be replaced with cream or goat cheese if not available. Adding a lot of dill makes this dish really come to life. The egg on top is a salute to the classic.

1. FOR PASTA, in a large skillet, bring cream to a boil over medium heat. Stir in 2 tablespoons of Boursin cheese. Reduce heat to low. Add cooked spaghetti and dill. Stir to combine. Stir in avocado oil. Season to taste with salt. Keep warm while preparing eggs.

2. FOR EGGS, in a small nonstick skillet, melt 2 teaspoons of butter over medium heat. Crack one egg into the hot pan, being careful not to break the yolk. Cook for 2–2½ minutes or until whites are cooked, but yolk is still runny. Transfer to a plate and repeat with remaining 3 eggs.

3. TO SERVE, divide pasta evenly among 4 plates. Top with fried egg and remaining boursin cheese if desired. Serve immediately.

SERVINGS: 4 | SOURCE: Little Rusted Ladle

½ cup heavy cream, optional

½ cup boursin or goat cheese, divided

4 cups spaghetti noodles, cooked

2 Tbsp. chopped fresh dill

2 Tbsp. avocado oil

Kosher salt to taste

2 Tbsp. unsalted butter, divided

4 medium eggs

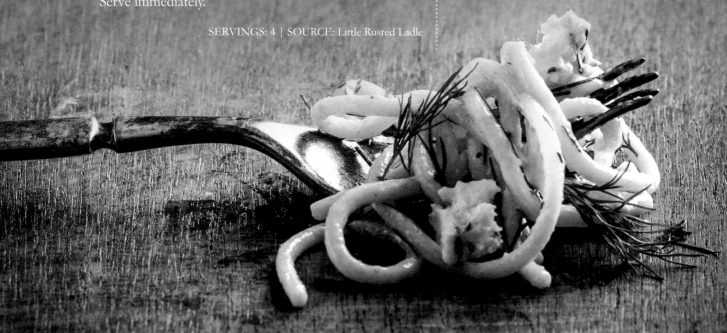

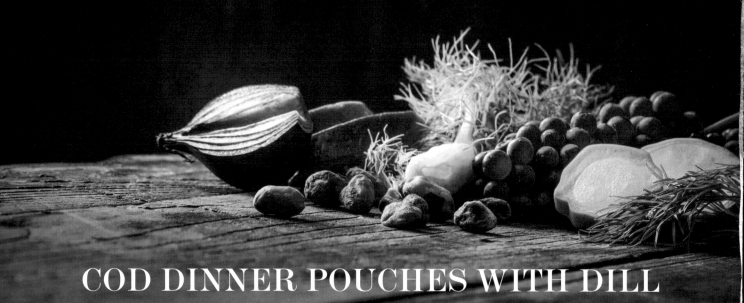

COD DINNER POUCHES WITH DILL

Cod is delicious when steamed in parchment paper. Adding fresh dill, vegetables, and quinoa make it something special. The quinoa cooks in the pouch with the vegetables making it a complete meal. Sprinkle fresh dill, pistachios, and champagne grapes over the top and you have a meal fit for royalty. Champagne grapes are available for a few weeks in early fall. Red or black seedless grapes may be substituted for the champagne grapes.

1. FOR DILL BUTTER, combine butter and next 5 ingredients in a small bowl. Set aside.

2. FOR COD POUCHES, preheat oven to 350 degrees. Brush one side of parchment squares with prepared dill butter. Place squash, zucchini, red onions, and quinoa evenly in the middle of each parchment square. Brush cod pieces generously with remaining dill butter. Place cod pieces on top of vegetables. Bring up sides of parchment paper, then pour 1 oz. broth over fish. Season with salt and pepper. Tie string around parchment paper, creating a pouch. Place pouches on a sheet pan. Bake for 18–20 minutes or until fish is cooked through. Serve by opening fish at the table, and garnish with fresh dill, pistachios and champagne grapes as desired.

1 stick unsalted butter, melted
½ cup fresh dill, loosely packed and chopped
2 Tbsp. fresh fennel fronds, chopped
½ tsp. kosher salt
½ tsp. freshly ground black pepper
2 tbsp. pickle juice
1 cup yellow squash, sliced
1 cup zucchini, sliced
2 ea. red pearl onions, peeled, cut into strips
½ cup quinoa, uncooked
4 squares parchment paper (15 X 12 in.)
4 pieces fresh cod (5–6 oz. each)
4 pieces of string (6-8 in. long)
½ cup vegetable broth
¼ cup champagne grapes, optional
Fresh dill for garnish, optional
2 Tbsp. roasted pistachio nuts, optional

SERVINGS: 4 | SOURCE: Little Rusted Ladle

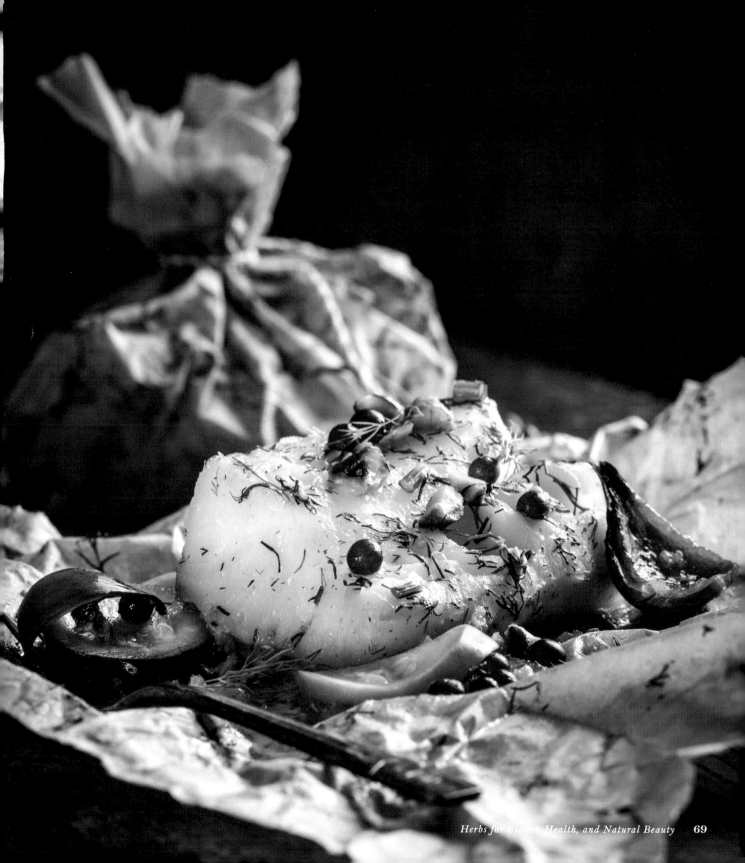

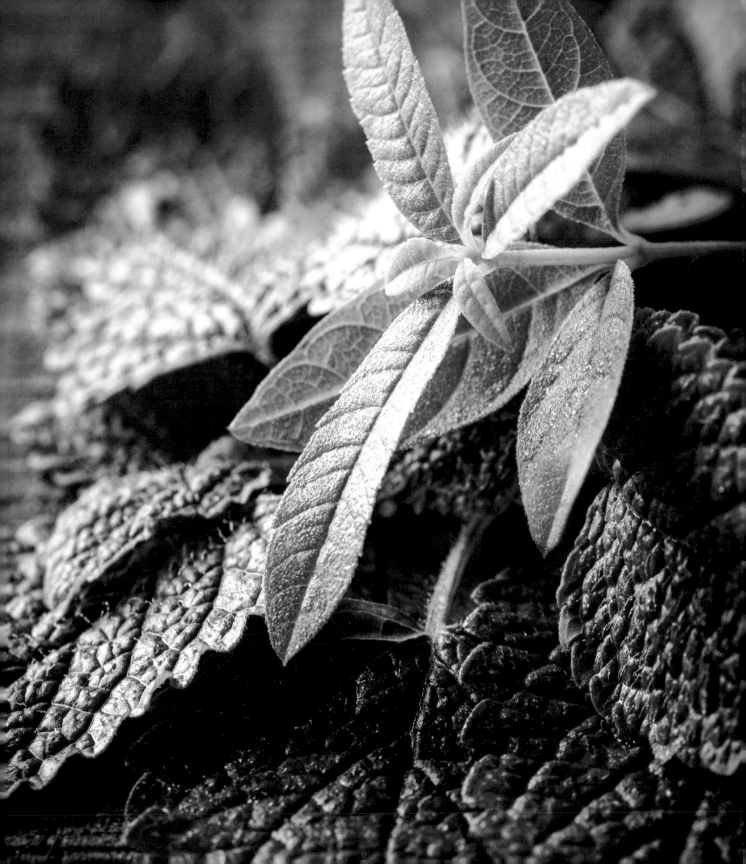

Chapter 6:
LEMON BALM
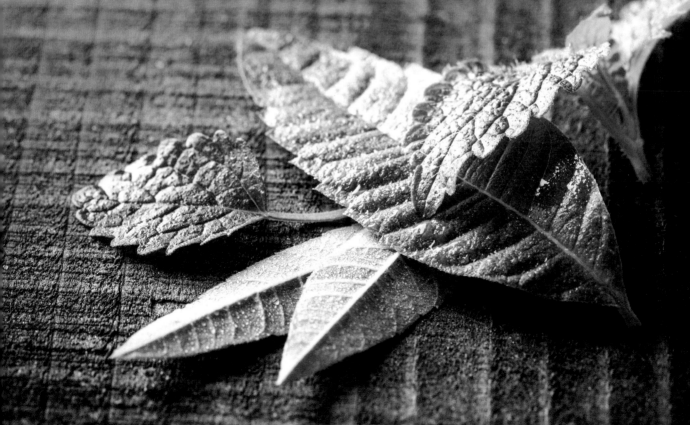 VERBENA

*T*here are very few herbs that create such an overwhelming sense of joy within me than fresh lemon balm or verbena. Rubbing the leaves of these herbs in my hands while breathing in deeply relaxes me like no other herb, except maybe rosemary. Research suggests that this is not an isolated response. As a matter of fact, lemon balm is linked to many health benefits including its ability to increase alertness, sharpen memory, and aid in restful sleep. It is used extensively in aromatherapy, perfumes, and lotions. That doesn't include any of the incredible culinary uses, which range from sauces and dressings to drinks and desserts. The mild lemony flavor of lemon balm leaves is a great addition to salads as well. Although this herb can take over a garden if allowed to do so, its benefits can help you forget how obnoxious it can be when it invades your flower beds.

LEMON BALM HUMMUS

This super easy appetizer dip is a great way to use up some of the lemon balm in your garden that can sometimes get overwhelming.

....

1 garlic clove

1 (1½ cups) can chickpeas, drained, rinsed

¼ cup tahini paste or sesame seed paste

1 avocado, chopped

1 cup fresh lemon balm leaves

¼ cup extra virgin olive oil

½ tsp. kosher salt

¼ cup fresh lime juice

1. In the bowl of a food processor, add garlic. Process until minced. Add remaining ingredients. Process until smooth. Serve with fresh vegetables, pita bread, or crackers.

SERVINGS: 4 | SOURCE: Little Rusted Ladle

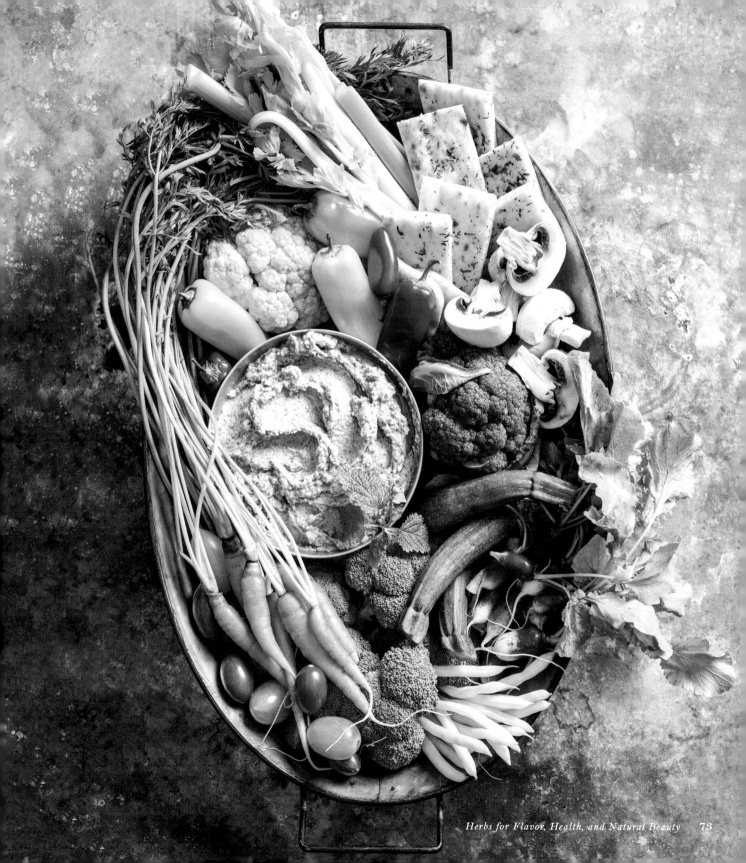

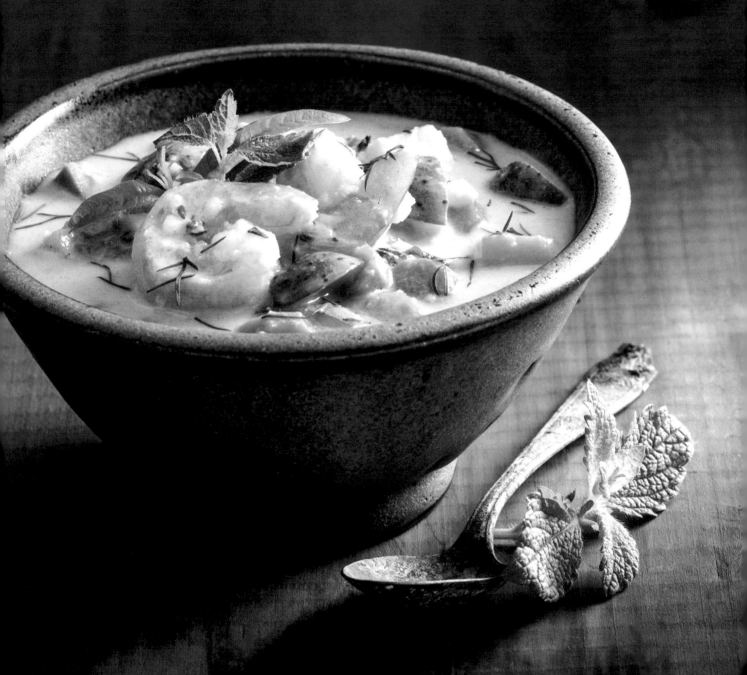

Nothing says east coast like seafood chowder. In this version, the lemon balm leaves take the place of spinach. By adding whole leaves at the end, the flavor stays intact, allowing for maximum lemon flavor. Of course, adding additional herbs such as thyme, dill, and tarragon add layers of flavor to this decadent soup.

LEMONY SEAFOOD CHOWDER

1 Tbsp. unsalted butter

1 Tbsp. extra virgin olive oil

¾ cup chopped onion

½ cup chopped celery

½ cup sliced carrots

3 small red potatoes, cubed

1 small sweet potato, cubed

2 garlic cloves, minced

3 Tbsp. unbleached flour

1½ cup seafood stock

1½ cup whole milk, divided

8 oz. fresh cod (1 cup), cut into 1-inch pieces

10 small shrimp, peeled, deveined

3 oz. lobster meat, cut into pieces

4 large sea scallops (3 ozs.), halved

3 Tbsp. fresh herbs (thyme, dill, and tarragon), chopped

½ cup fresh lemon balm leaves

1. In a medium saucepan over medium heat, melt butter with olive oil. Add onion and next five ingredients. Sauté for 4–5 minutes or until softened. Add flour and cook 4–5 minutes, stirring often.

2. Add stock and remaining milk to vegetables. Bring to a simmer. Cook for 10–15 minutes or until potatoes are almost cooked through and soup has thickened.

3. Stir in cod and next 4 ingredients. Cook an additional 5–7 minutes or until seafood is barely cooked through. Add lemon balm leaves and serve.

SERVINGS: 4 | SOURCE: Little Rusted Ladle

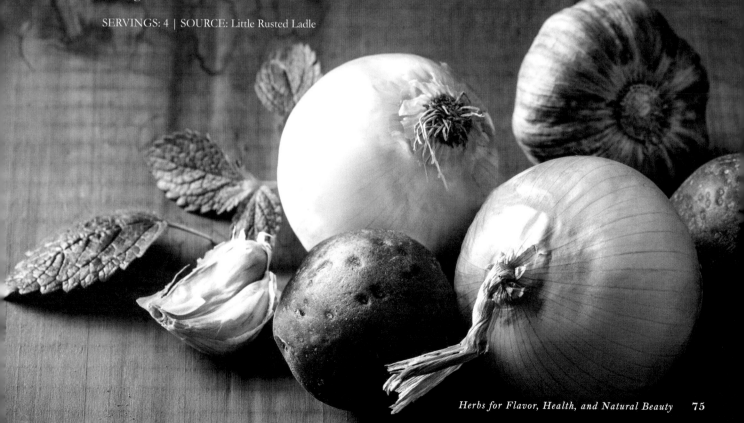

LEMON BALM PASTA SALAD

Lemon balm acts both as a flavoring and as a greens replacement in this refreshing pasta salad. Goat cheese adds an added tang to the taste buds and the maple-glazed pistachios add sweetness and that needed crunch to make this salad tasty on so many levels. You can substitute any pasta you wish for the tri-colored pasta used in the photo. Lemon verbena may be substituted for the lemon balm.

½ cup pistachios, shelled and roasted

2 Tbsp. maple syrup

¼ tsp. red pepper flakes

½ tsp. kosher salt

2 cups multi-colored pasta, cooked, rinsed, and lightly oiled

3 Tbsp. light olive oil

1 Tbsp. apple cider vinegar

1 Tbsp. honey

2 tsp. deli-style mustard

1 cup fresh lemon balm leaves

¼ cup crumbled goat cheese

Fresh cracked black pepper to taste

1. FOR GLAZED PISTACHIOS, toast pistachios in a small skillet over medium heat. Add maple syrup and red pepper flakes. Cook for 1–2 minutes or until maple syrup has thickened and nuts are glazed. Transfer to a sheet pan lined with parchment paper and cool completely. Break up nuts and set aside.

2. FOR DRESSING, in a small mason jar with a screw top lid, combine olive oil, and next three ingredients. Shake vigorously until thickened. Set aside.

3. TO MAKE PASTA SALAD, in a medium size bowl, toss together cooked pasta and remaining ingredients. Add dressing and toss to coat. Top with glazed pistachios and serve.

SERVINGS: 4 | SOURCE: Little Rusted Ladle

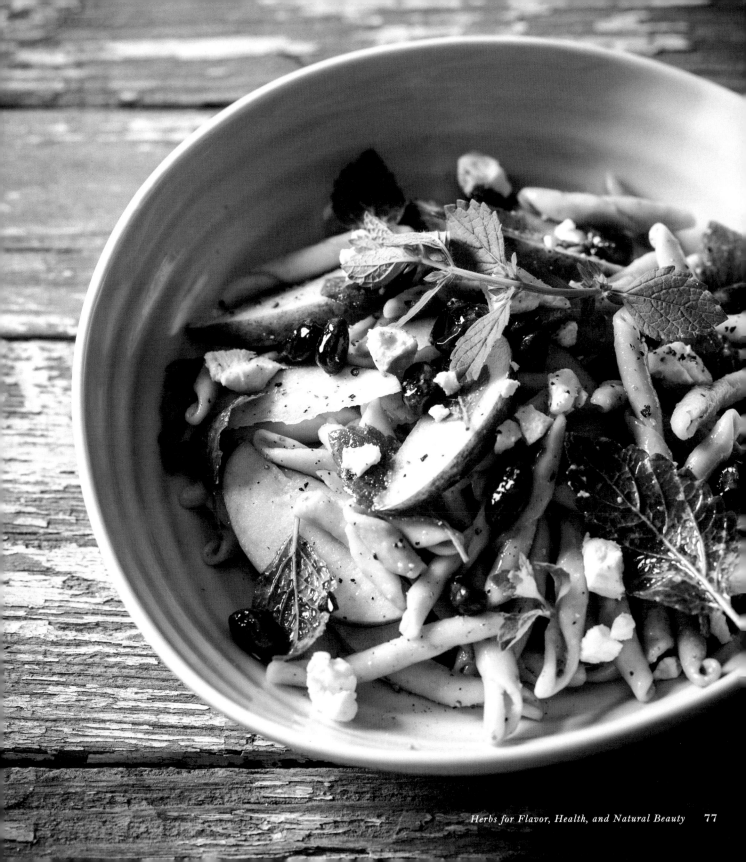

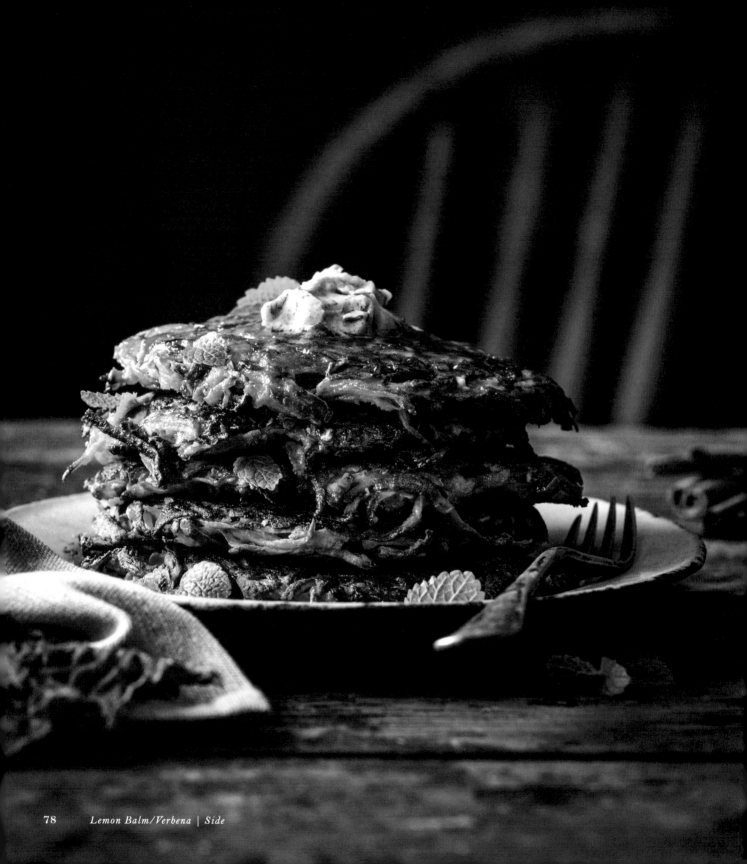

SWEET POTATO CAKES WITH LEMON BALM JAVA BUTTER

Sweet potatoes work well shredded and used as cakes similar to latkes (potato pancakes). The lemon balm is this recipe is used in in the cakes, the butter, and sprinkled on top. The flavors of coffee and cinnamon in the butter add a uniquely bold flavor that complement these lemony, sweet cakes really well. Enjoy them as a side with fish, roasted turkey, or barbecued meats.

2 large eggs, beaten

¼ cup unbleached flour

2 Tbsp. unsalted butter, melted

4 cups shredded sweet potatoes

¼ cup fresh chives, chopped

½ cup fresh lemon balm leaves, roughly chopped

½ tsp. kosher salt

¼ tsp. turmeric

1 garlic clove, minced

1 Tbsp. vegetable oil

1 stick unsalted butter, softened

½ tsp. cinnamon

2 Tbsp. brown sugar

1 tsp. instant coffee granules

2 Tbsp. finely chopped lemon balm leaves

Fresh lemon balm leaves, for garnish, optional

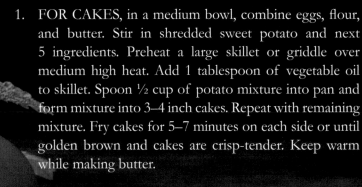

1. FOR CAKES, in a medium bowl, combine eggs, flour, and butter. Stir in shredded sweet potato and next 5 ingredients. Preheat a large skillet or griddle over medium high heat. Add 1 tablespoon of vegetable oil to skillet. Spoon ½ cup of potato mixture into pan and form mixture into 3–4 inch cakes. Repeat with remaining mixture. Fry cakes for 5–7 minutes on each side or until golden brown and cakes are crisp-tender. Keep warm while making butter.

2. FOR LEMON BALM JAVA BUTTER, in a small bowl, combine 1 stick butter and next four ingredients. Stir until smooth. Serve butter over warm cakes with fresh lemon balm leaves for garnish.

SERVINGS: 4 | SOURCE: Little Rusted Ladle

LEMON VERBENA CHICKEN DRUMMIES

Lemon verbena has a wonderful lemon flavor that works extremely well when placed under the skin of roasted chicken drumsticks. The additional herb butter will keep the chicken juicy while adding incredible flavor.

....

1 Tbsp. fresh lemon basil leaves, chopped

1 Tbsp. fresh thyme leaves (lemon or lime)

1 Tbsp. chopped fresh chives

2 garlic cloves, minced

½ tsp. fresh ground black pepper

1 tsp. kosher salt

4 Tbsp. unsalted butter, softened

8 chicken drumsticks

½ cup fresh lemon verbena leaves, loosely packed

½ tsp. paprika, optional

1. Combine lemon basil and next six ingredients in a small bowl. Stir until herbs are well blended into butter.

2. Take one drumstick in your hands. Starting from the wide end, work your fingers between the skin and the meat making a pocket. Work about a teaspoon of the reserved herb butter under the skin of the chicken. Place 2–3 lemon verbena leaves in between the skin and the meat. Pull skin up and over the leaves. Secure with toothpicks. Repeat with remaining drumsticks.

3. Sprinkle with paprika. Bake at 350 degrees for one hour or until juices run clear. Serve garnished with fresh herbs.

SERVINGS: 4 | SOURCE: Little Rusted Ladle

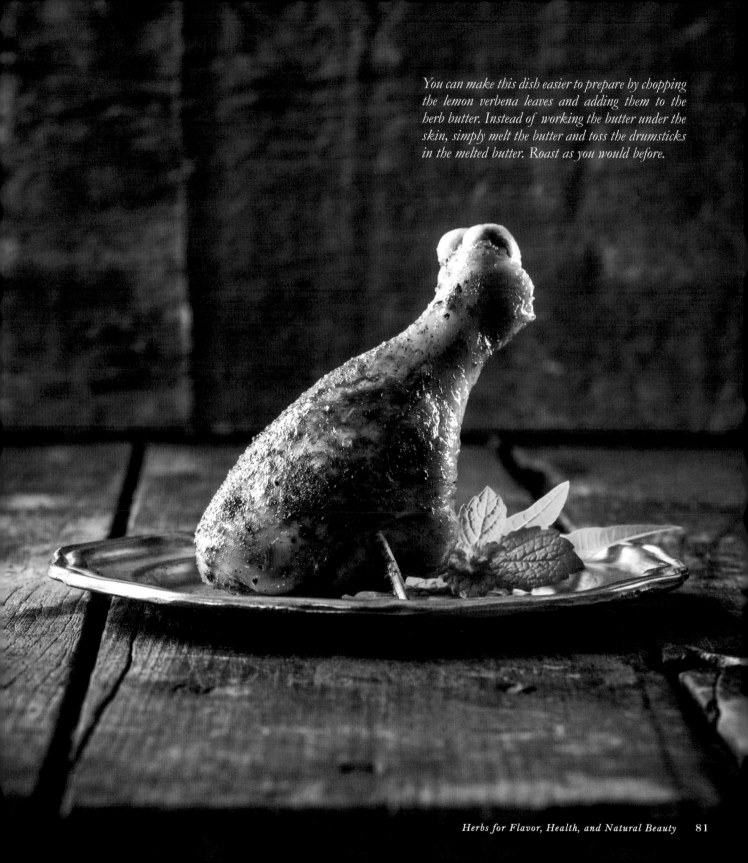

You can make this dish easier to prepare by chopping the lemon verbena leaves and adding them to the herb butter. Instead of working the butter under the skin, simply melt the butter and toss the drumsticks in the melted butter. Roast as you would before.

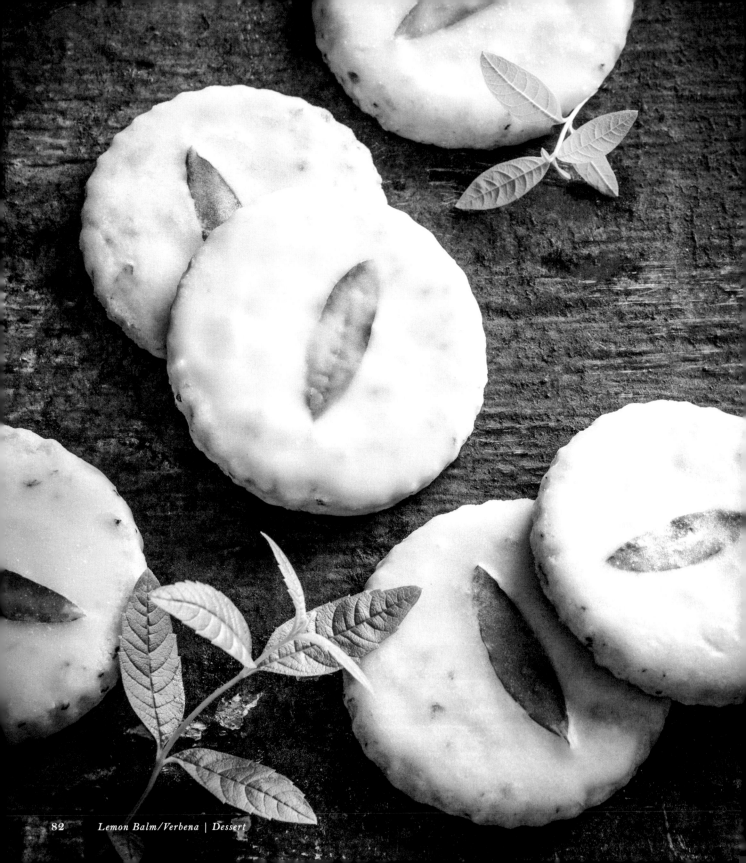

LEMON VERBENA SHORTBREAD COOKIES

These delightful shortbread cookies get their refreshing flavor from lemon verbena. By using a leaf as a decoration under the glaze, you add a nice finishing touch visually while also adding more lemon flavor. For a more consistent look, cut the circles into perfect rounds with a 2-inch round cutter.

1¾ cup powdered sugar, divided

2 sticks unsalted butter, softened

1 tsp. salt

2 cups unbleached flour

⅓ cup chopped lemon verbena or lemon balm leaves

2 tsp. meringue powder, optional

2 Tbsp. lemonade, prepared

12 lemon verbena or lemon balm leaves

1. Combine ¾ cup powdered sugar and next four ingredients in the bowl of a food processor. Process until dough forms. Transfer mixture to a piece of parchment paper and form into a log about 2 inches in diameter. Refrigerate four hours.

2. Preheat oven to 350 degrees. Cut dough log crosswise into ½-inch slices. Place slices 2–3 inches apart onto a sheet pan lined with parchment paper. Bake for 30–35 minutes or until lightly browned on top. Cool cookies on wire rack.

3. While cookies are cooling, make glaze by combining remaining 1 cup powdered sugar, meringue powder, and lemonade in a small bowl until smooth. Place one lemon verbena or lemon balm leaf in the center of each cookie. Pour about 1 tablespoon of glaze over each cookie. Turn each cookie to let glaze cover top completely. Let dry completely on wire racks. Store in containers.

SERVINGS: 12 | SOURCE: Little Rusted Ladle

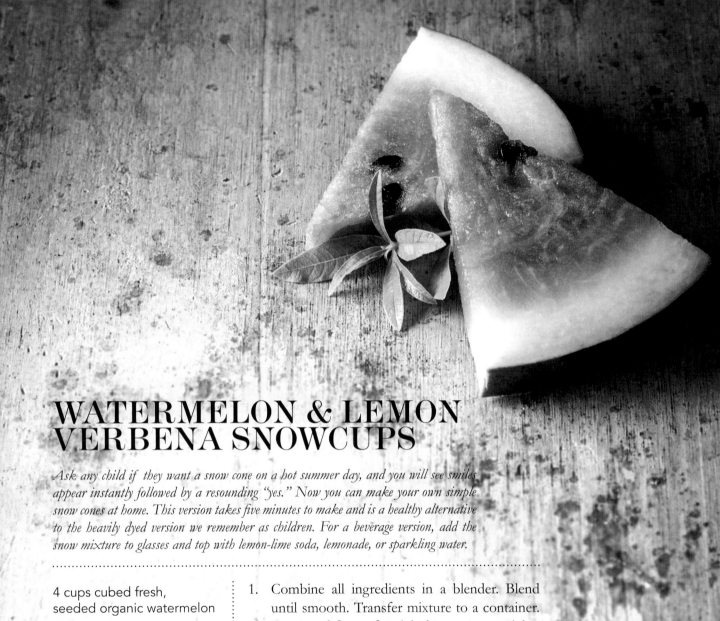

WATERMELON & LEMON VERBENA SNOWCUPS

Ask any child if they want a snow cone on a hot summer day, and you will see smiles appear instantly followed by a resounding "yes." Now you can make your own simple snow cones at home. This version takes five minutes to make and is a healthy alternative to the heavily dyed version we remember as children. For a beverage version, add the snow mixture to glasses and top with lemon-lime soda, lemonade, or sparkling water.

4 cups cubed fresh, seeded organic watermelon

¼ cup sugar or honey

1 cup lemon verbena leaves, loosely packed

1 Tbsp. fresh lime juice

½ tsp. fine sea salt

1. Combine all ingredients in a blender. Blend until smooth. Transfer mixture to a container. Cover and freeze for eight hours or overnight.

2. TO SERVE, use a metal spoon or ice cream spade to scrape the top of the frozen mixture across the top, creating a layer of watermelon snow. Spoon mixture into cups and eat immediately or freeze mixture until needed.

SERVINGS: 4 | SOURCE: Little Rusted Ladle

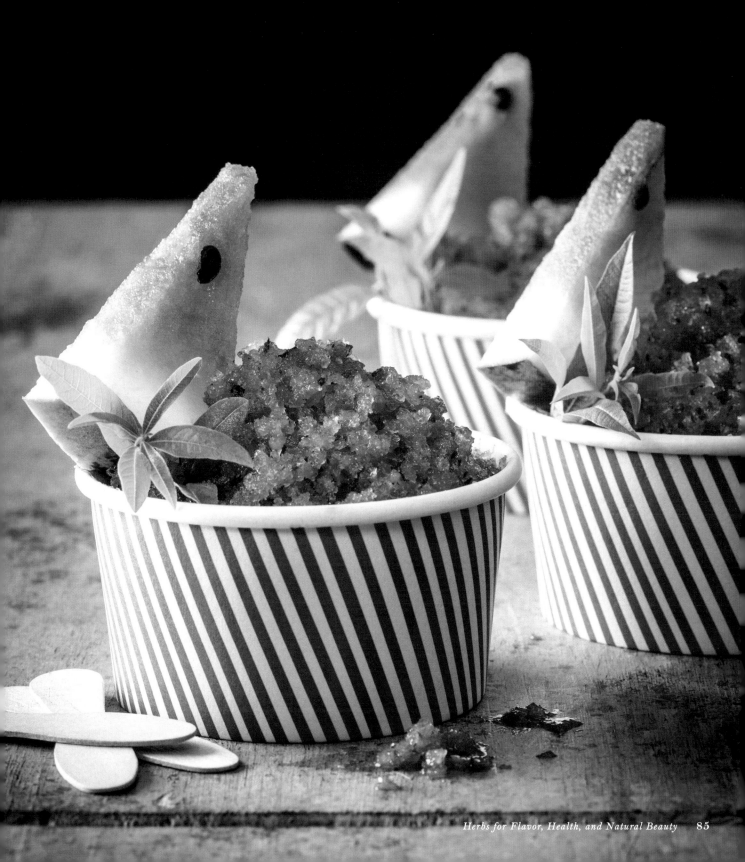

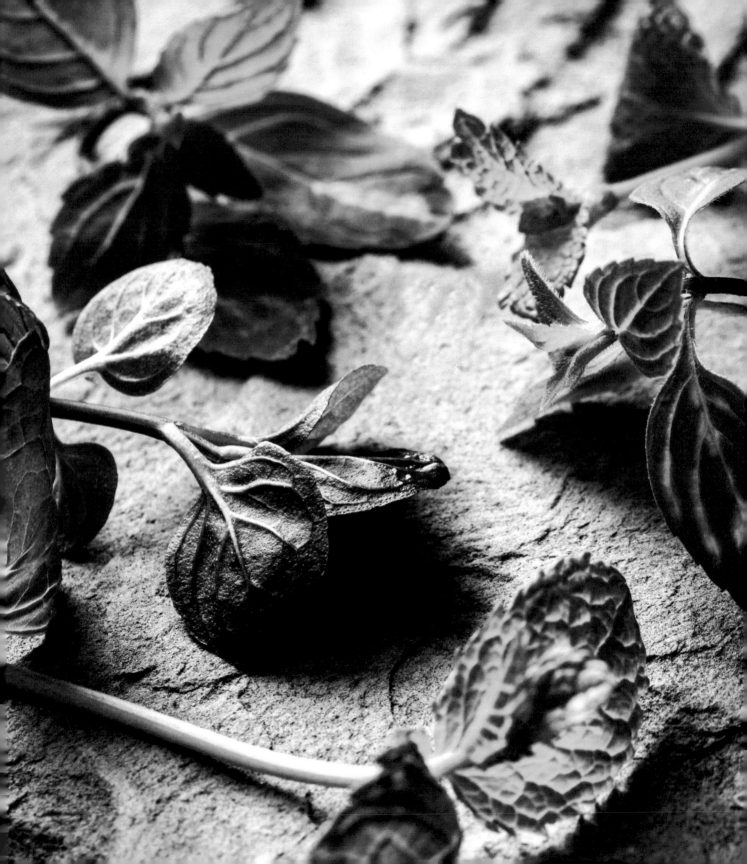

Chapter 7:
MINT

Mint is known for being added to chocolates, candy, and, of course, mouthwash and toothpaste. However, mint has a lot more going for it than those common uses. Did you know that mint is used to help stomach ailments, headaches, and nausea? It is also pretty fantastic as an addition to beverages. Mint also makes a great addition to marinades, dressings, dips, and salsas. The varieties of mint are so plentiful that you can find a different mint for just about every use. From the ever popular spearmint and peppermint to lesser-known varieties like chocolate and ginger mint, this powerhouse herb will make your culinary and beauty creations ones to remember.

SEARED SEA SCALLOPS WITH MINT & PEA PUREE

When seared sea scallops are infused and flavored with fresh mint and farm fresh peas, it creates a combination of flavors that is just plain delicious. I recommend using the freshest, largest diver sea scallops you can find. You can substitute shrimp for the scallops if they are not available in your area.

1 cup vegetable broth or water

1 cup fresh or frozen peas

¼ cup greek yogurt

1 cup fresh mint leaves, loosely packed

Salt and pepper to taste

5 jumbo sea scallops (u10)

5 small fresh mint leaves

½ Tbsp. unsalted butter

½ Tbsp. extra virgin olive oil

1. FOR MINT AND PEA PUREE, in a small saucepan, bring broth to a simmer over medium heat. Add peas and cook for 3–4 minutes or until crisp-tender. Add peas and liquid to a blender with greek yogurt and mint. Blend until smooth. Transfer to a small bowl. Season with salt and pepper to taste. Set aside.

2. FOR SCALLOPS, using a sharp knife, make ¼-inch deep cuts in a grid pattern on one side of each scallop. Press one mint leaf onto one side of each scallop. Season with salt and pepper. Preheat a medium skillet over medium-high heat. Add butter and olive oil. When butter has melted completely, add scallops mint-side down. Sear scallops for 1–2 minutes or until golden brown. Turn scallops over using a pair of tongs. Cook an additional 1–2 minutes or until just cooked through. Transfer to a plate and let rest while preparing plate.

3. TO SERVE, spoon 5 dollops of reserved puree onto a warm plate. Place one scallop onto each dollop of puree. Garnish with fresh mint. Serve.

SERVINGS: 4 | SOURCE: Little Rusted Ladle

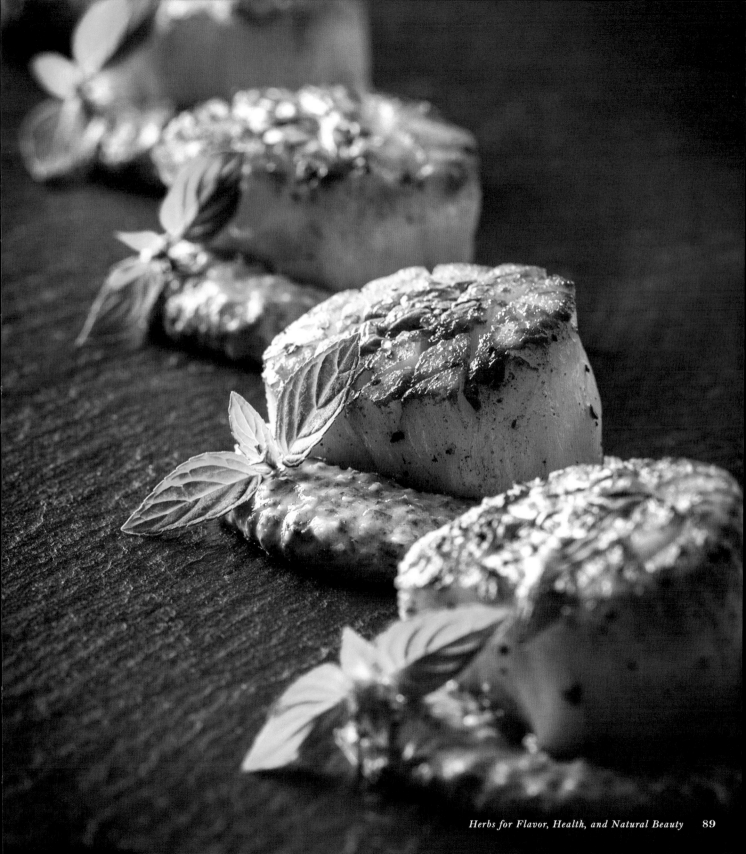

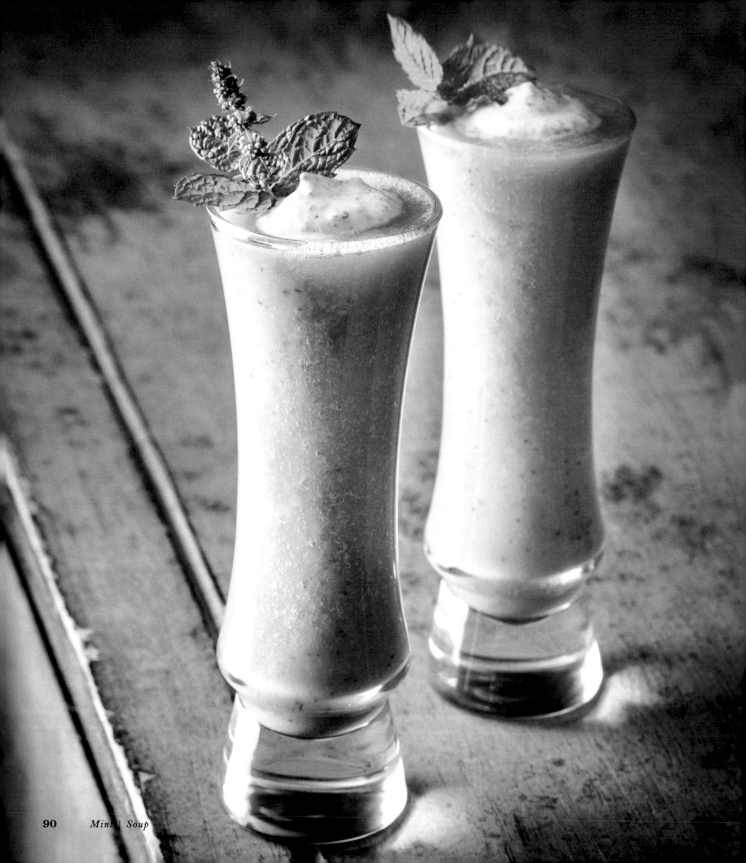

DOUBLE MELON SOUP SHOOTERS WITH GINGER MINT CREAM

Melon tastes great on its own or in drinks. This recipe uses two melon flavors combined in one fresh soup. The mint cream adds a nice balance of acidity to the sweetness of the melon.

....

2 cups cubed honeydew melon

½ cup seedless cucumber, peeled, seeded, and cubed

½ cup chopped avocado

1 Tbsp. fresh lime juice

½ cup fresh spearmint leaves, loosely packed

2 cups cubed cantaloupe

½ cup chopped fresh orange segments

1 cup greek yogurt

½ cup fresh ginger mint leaves, loosely packed, finely chopped

1 tsp. grated fresh ginger

1 Tbsp. honey

1. Combine honeydew and next four ingredients in a blender. Blend until smooth. Transfer to a pourable container. Cover and refrigerate until ready to serve.

2. Clean blender, then add cantaloupe and orange. Blend until smooth. Transfer to another pourable container. Cover and refrigerate until ready to serve.

3. IN A SMALL BOWL, combine yogurt, mint, ginger, and honey until well blended. Refrigerate until ready to serve.

4. TO SERVE, holding one fruit mixture in each hand, pour at the same time into small glasses until almost full. Spoon a tablespoon of ginger mint cream on top and garnish with a sprig of fresh mint. Serve.

SERVINGS: 4
SOURCE: Little Rusted Ladle

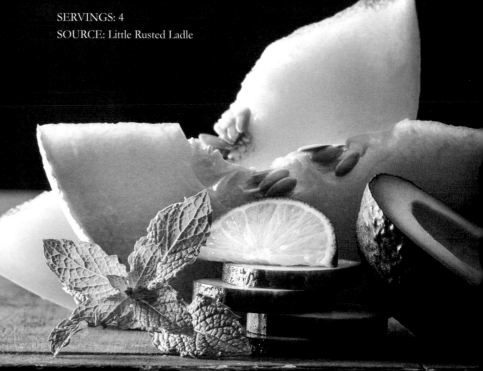

CARROT & MINT SALAD WITH CRUNCHY WHEAT BERRIES

The beauty of peeled carrots is really dramatic in this salad when you add yellow and red carrot peelings as well. These carrots are increasingly more common in local grocery and health food stores around the country. Crunchy wheat berries add great flavor and texture to this salad. The star is really the mint and the flavor it adds to this normally boring vegetable. A light vinaigrette brings all the flavors together. If the wheat berries seem like too much hassle, simply omit them.

¼ cup wheat berries, rinsed, optional

¾ cup water

¼ cup vegetable oil, divided

¼ cup sunflower seeds

1 cup fresh mint leaves, divided

½ tsp. toasted sesame oil

½ tsp. kosher salt

3 large carrots (1 orange, 1 yellow, 1 red)

Cold water

1 Tbsp. rice wine vinegar

2 Tbsp. honey

1 thai chili pepper, finely chopped

Salt

1. FOR WHEAT BERRIES, place berries in a small saucepan. Cover with water. Cover pan and cook over medium heat until water boils. Reduce heat to simmer and cook for one hour. Drain berries well and transfer to a plate lined with paper towels. Dry berries completely. In a small skillet, heat oil over medium heat until hot. Add berries and fry for about 1 minute or until crunchy on the outside. With a slotted spoon, transfer berries to paper towels. Reserve 2 tablespoons of oil for dressing. In a small bowl, combine sunflower seeds, half of the mint leaves, toasted sesame oil, kosher salt, and fried wheat berries. Toss to combine and set aside.

2. FOR SALAD, using a vegetable peeler, peel carrots continually until carrots are too small to peel. Transfer carrot peels to a medium size bowl. Cover with cold water. Refrigerate for one hour or until carrots have firmed up. Drain carrots well, removing as much water as possible. In a small bowl, combine rice wine vinegar, honey, chili pepper, salt, and reserved 2 tablespoons of oil. Whisk to combine. Add to bowl of carrots. Toss to coat. Add crunchy wheat berry mixture and remaining mint leaves. Serve.

SERVINGS: 4 | SOURCE: Little Rusted Ladle

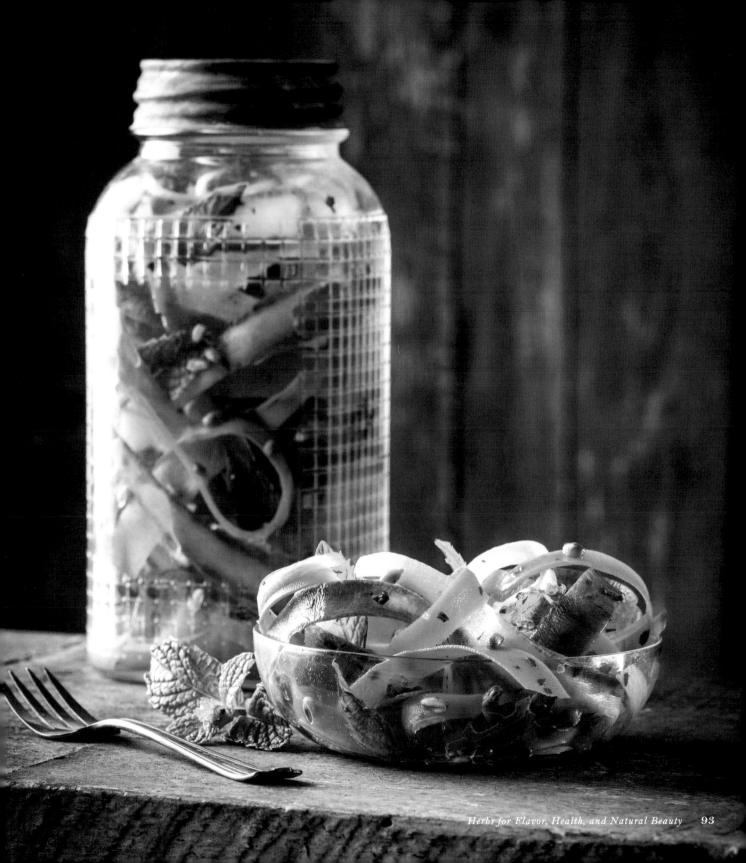

¾ cup fresh mint
leaves, divided

1 tbsp. tamari gluten-free,
reduced-sodium soy sauce

1 Tbsp. chili garlic sauce

1 Tbsp. honey

2 Tbsp. rice vinegar

½ tsp. toasted sesame oil

½ tsp. curry powder

3 Tbsp. peanut or vegetable oil

8 oz. fresh tuna steak,
cut into 4 pieces

1½ cups rice noodles,
cooked, rinsed with cold water

1 cup shredded broccoli

1 cup chopped romanesco

½ cup thinly sliced red onion

½ cup thinly sliced shiitake
mushrooms, stems removed

1 Tbsp. chopped lemon
verbena leaves

2 english cucumbers,
peeled into long strips

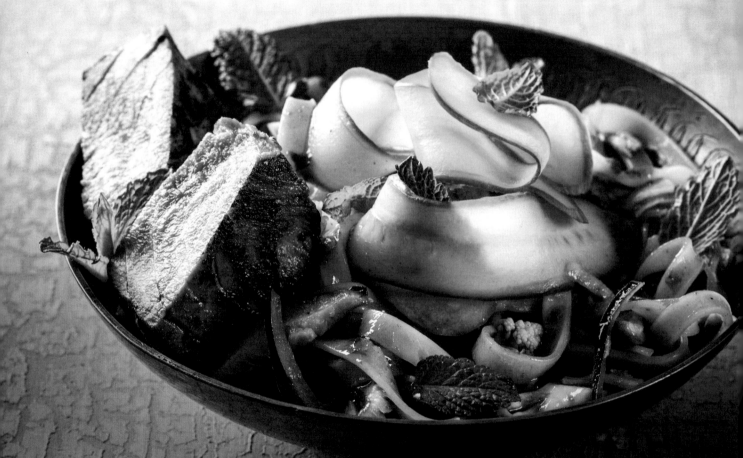

*If rare tuna isn't your preference, simply cook the tuna a little longer on each side.
Tamara is found in the asian section of most grocery stores. You can substitute
low-sodium soy sauce if desired. If you plan on making this salad ahead of time,
double the dressing. The pasta has a tendency to absorb the dressing the longer it sits.*

THAI NOODLE SALAD WITH MINT & SEARED TUNA

Mint is a staple in thai food and for good reason. This salad is no exception. The mint adds a wonderful freshness and flavor to the dish, once for the dressing, then at the end in the salad. The seared tuna adds some sophistication. You are welcome to substitute cooked shrimp or chicken to this dish or have it without protein if you would prefer to keep it light.

1. FOR CHILE MINT VINAIGRETTE, finely chop ¼ cup of the mint leaves and add to an 8-ounce jar. Add tamari sauce and next six ingredients. Cover jar with lid and shake vigorously until thickened. Transfer 3 tablespoons of the dressing to a small plate, and refrigerate the remainder until ready to serve.

2. FOR THE TUNA, add tuna pieces to plate with dressing and turn all sides until tuna is well-coated with dressing. Cover and refrigerate for 1–2 hours, turning fish after 30 minutes. Preheat a medium nonstick skillet over medium-high heat. Add 1 teaspoon of oil to the pan. Remove as much dressing as possible from the tuna, then add to the hot skillet. Cook for 30 seconds, then turn again over using a pair of tongs. Repeat until all sides are seared. Transfer seared tuna to a plate, cut pieces in half, and set aside until ready to assemble salad. Tuna should be rare in the center.

3. TO ASSEMBLE SALAD, combine cooked rice noodles and next six ingredients, including remaining ½ cup of mint leaves, in a medium size bowl. Add prepared dressing and toss to coat. Serve topped with 2–3 slices of cucumber and two pieces of seared tuna. Enjoy.

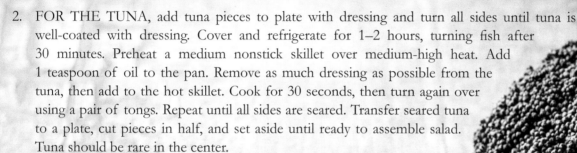

SERVINGS: 4
SOURCE: Little Rusted Ladle

RACK OF LAMB WITH MINT PESTO

Mint and lamb are best friends. Both enhance and compliment the flavor of the other. The pesto for this recipe is made with walnuts and herbs to help balance and increase the complexity of the finished dish. Frenched racks simply means exposing the bones halfway down. They are more readily available in grocery stores these days. If they are not available, ask your butcher if they can french the lamb racks for you to save time.

2 cups fresh mint leaves, loosely packed

¼ cup walnut pieces, toasted

2 garlic cloves, minced

1 Tbsp. fresh lemon juice

1 cup fresh herbs (parsley, lemon verbena, chives), chopped

½ cup extra virgin olive oil

2 racks Lamb (1¼ 1½ lbs. ea.), frenched

Salt and pepper

1. FOR PESTO, in a food processor bowl, add mint and next four ingredients. While running processor, slowly add olive oil until mixture is smooth. Transfer to a bowl.

2. FOR LAMB, season lamb racks with salt and pepper and let rest at room temperature for 20–30 minutes. Preheat a large skillet over medium-high heat. Sear lamb racks on all sides until well browned, about 10 minutes. Place lamb racks on a sheet pan with sides. Brush lamb with half of prepared pesto. Roast in a 400 degree oven for 20 minutes or until lamb reaches 120 degrees. Let stand covered for 10 minutes. Serve with remaining mint pesto on the side.

SERVINGS: 4 | SOURCE: Little Rusted Ladle

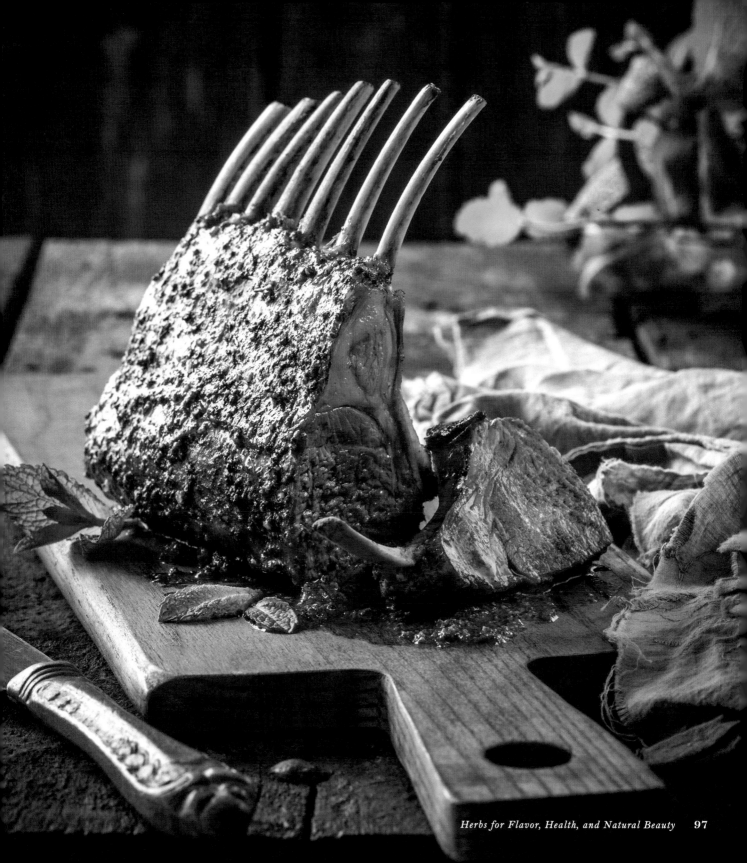

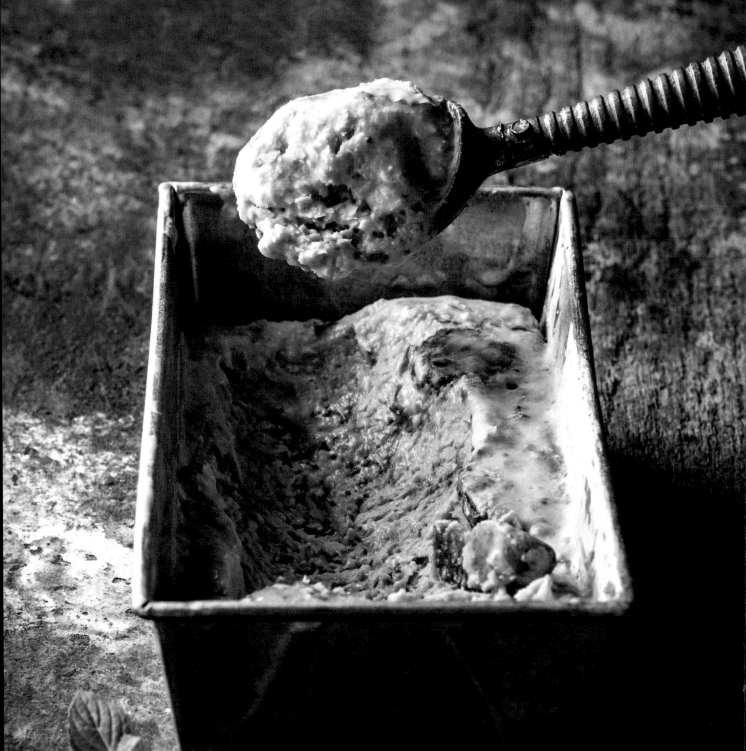

STRAWBERRY LEMON CREAM WITH MINT

This creamy summer treat is a great way to utilize strawberries when they are in season. Fresh mint adds a wonderful freshness that will put a smile on your kids' faces. For a smoother version, run the mixture through an ice cream machine before freezing the mixture.

1 cup heavy cream

½ cup sugar

½ cup fresh mint leaves, divided

2 Tbsp. fresh lemon juice

½ tsp. pure vanilla extract

1 cup hulled, sliced fresh strawberries

1. IN A SMALL SAUCEPAN, combine cream and sugar. Bring to a simmer, stirring often until sugar is dissolved. Remove pan from heat, and stir in half of mint leaves. Let mint steep in cream for ten minutes. Remove mint from cream with a fork.

2. Stir in remaining ingredients except remaining mint. Refrigerate mixture for one hour. Add remaining mint and stir mixture again. Cover and freeze until firm. When ready to serve, remove mixture from freezer and let soften at room temperature for 5–10 minutes. Scoop and enjoy.

SERVINGS: 4 | SOURCE: Little Rusted Ladle

MANGO MINT SMOOTHIE

Mango and mint are a match made in heaven. Especially when they are in the form of a refreshing smoothie. This recipe is so easy to make and so tasty. It is best tasting when you use mangoes in season. Simply peel, chop, and freeze the mangoes on foil-lined sheet pans, then place the pieces into small freezer bags.

1. Combine all ingredients except sprigs of fresh mint in a blender. Blend on high until smooth. Pour into glasses and serve. Garnish with a sprig of fresh mint.

SERVINGS: 4 | SOURCE: Little Rusted Ladle

2 cups cubed frozen mango

¾ cup pineapple flavored greek yogurt

¾ cup coconut milk

1 cup ice

¾ cup fresh orange juice

½ cup fresh spearmint leaves, washed

Sprigs fresh mint

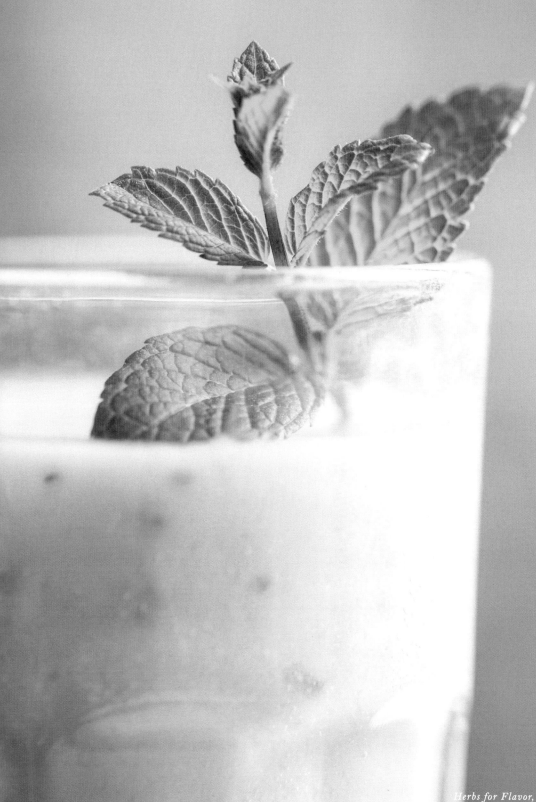

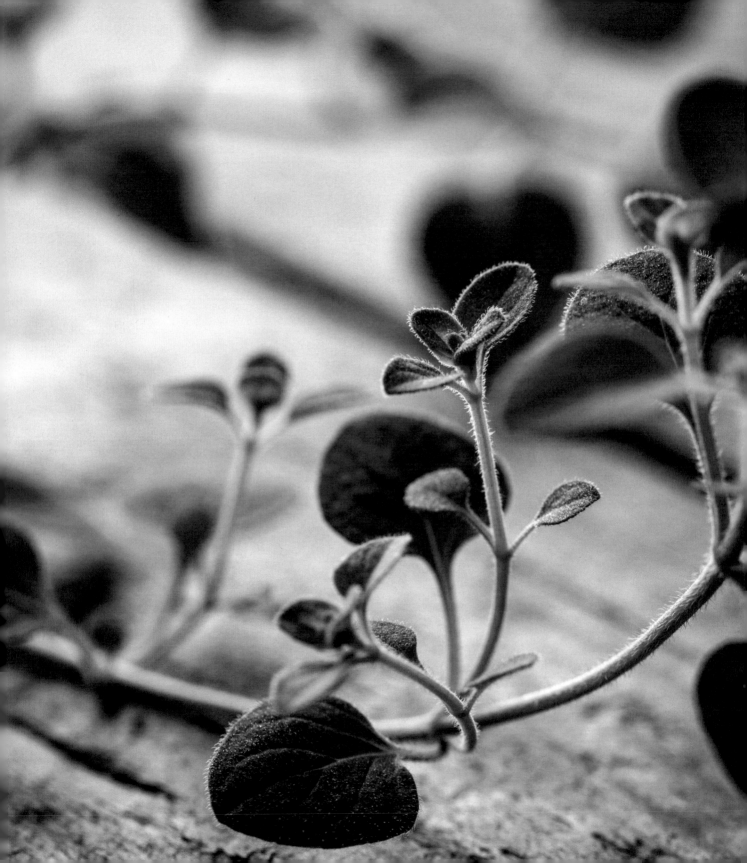

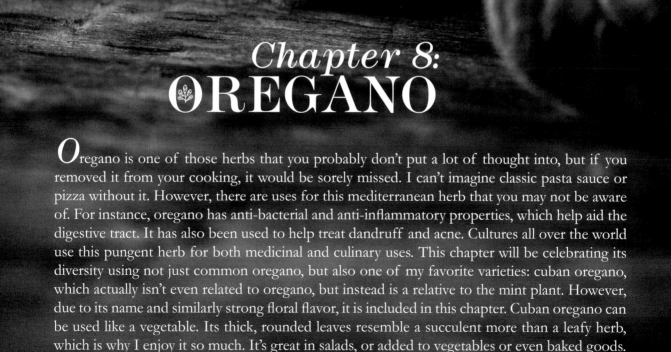

Chapter 8:
OREGANO

*O*regano is one of those herbs that you probably don't put a lot of thought into, but if you removed it from your cooking, it would be sorely missed. I can't imagine classic pasta sauce or pizza without it. However, there are uses for this mediterranean herb that you may not be aware of. For instance, oregano has anti-bacterial and anti-inflammatory properties, which help aid the digestive tract. It has also been used to help treat dandruff and acne. Cultures all over the world use this pungent herb for both medicinal and culinary uses. This chapter will be celebrating its diversity using not just common oregano, but also one of my favorite varieties: cuban oregano, which actually isn't even related to oregano, but instead is a relative to the mint plant. However, due to its name and similarly strong floral flavor, it is included in this chapter. Cuban oregano can be used like a vegetable. Its thick, rounded leaves resemble a succulent more than a leafy herb, which is why I enjoy it so much. It's great in salads, or added to vegetables or even baked goods.

ZA'ATAR FLATBREAD

This popular middle eastern seasoning gets its flavor from dried sumac, sesame seeds, oregano, and thyme. It is a lively combination that will wake up your taste buds. Sprinkle it on flatbread, yogurt, or just about anything else. For added oregano flavor, add fresh cuban oregano leaves with a red pepper olive and tomato spread for dipping.

2 Tbsp. sesame seeds

1 Tbsp. dried chopped oregano

1 tsp. dried chopped marjoram

1 tsp. kosher salt

1 Tbsp. chopped fresh greek oregano

1 Tbsp. chopped fresh cuban oregano

1 Tbsp. chopped fresh thyme leaves

2 Tbsp. ground sumac

½ tsp. ground cumin

2 greek-style flatbread

1 Tbsp. extra virgin olive oil

¼ tsp. ground black pepper

1. Toast sesame seeds in a small skillet over medium-low heat for about five minutes until golden brown. Add oregano and marjoram. Toast an additional minute. Remove from heat and let cool completely.

2. Grind sesame seed mixture, salt, and fresh herbs with a mortal and pestle until spices are ground and aromatic. Add ground sumac and cumin. Stir mixture and transfer to an airtight container until needed.

3. TO PREPARE FLATBREAD, brush both flatbreads with olive oil. Sprinkle prepared za'atar liberally over bread. Bake at 375 degrees for 5–7 minutes. Remove from oven, cut into wedges, and serve with lemon verbena hummus.

SERVINGS: 4 | SOURCE: Little Rusted Ladle

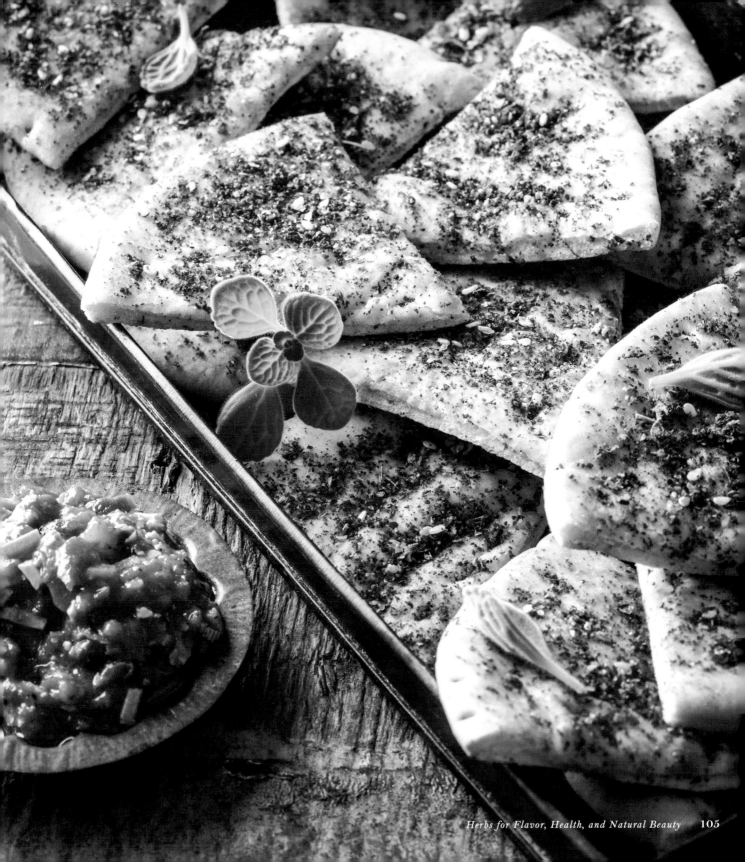

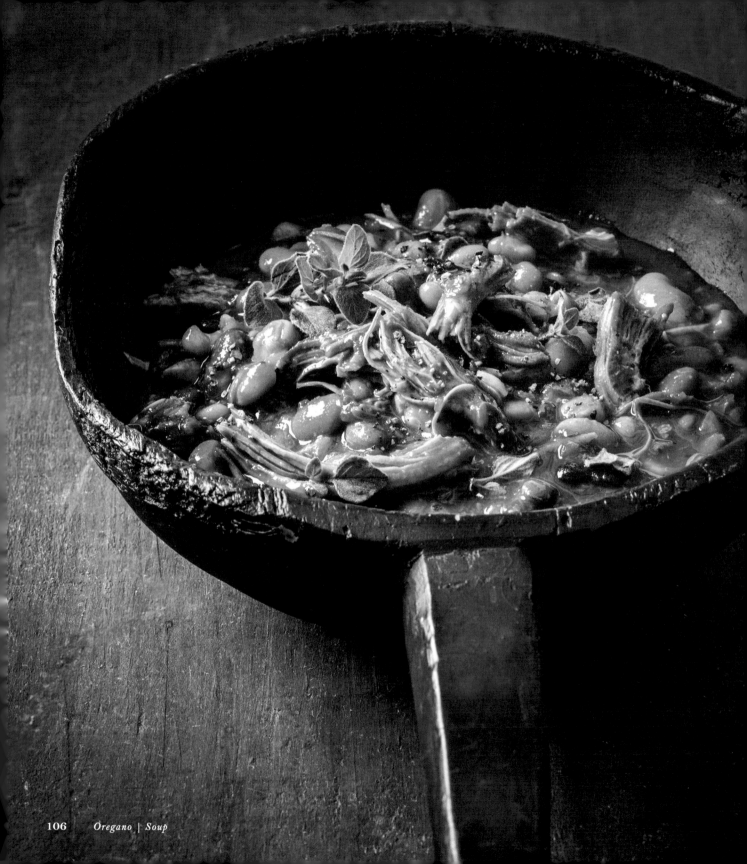

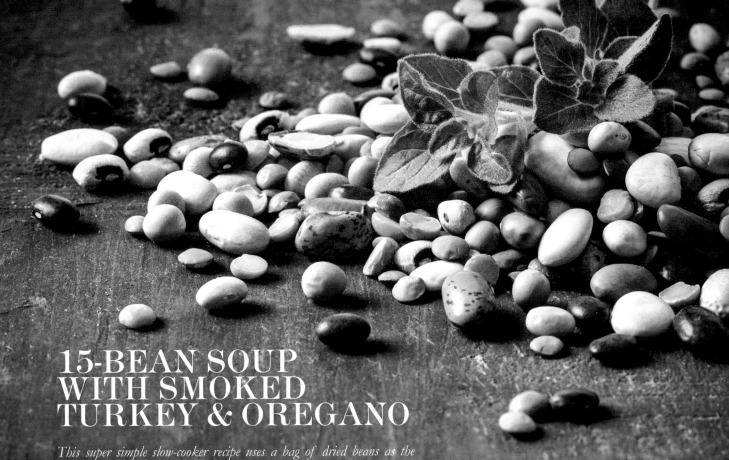

15-BEAN SOUP WITH SMOKED TURKEY & OREGANO

This super simple slow-cooker recipe uses a bag of dried beans as the base. I used smoked turkey from the grocery store for the meat, but feel free to substitute ham, sausage, or smoked brisket as well. The oregano really adds a wonderful flavor to this thick soup. After a hard days' work, there's nothing better than coming home to the smells of slow-cooked food.

There is a seasoning packet that comes with the beans. I did not use it for this recipe since I wanted to highlight the oregano, but feel free to add it if you wish. Serve it with warm, crusty bread slathered with butter.

1 (20 oz.) pkg. 15 bean soup mix, rinsed

4 cups water

4 cups chicken broth

1 cup diced onion

1 garlic clove, chopped

1 Tbsp. dried oregano

2 cups smoked turkey meat, pulled

1 can fire roasted diced tomatoes

½ cup fresh oregano leaves

Salt and pepper to taste

1. Transfer rinsed beans to a large bowl. Cover with water and soak overnight. Drain water and transfer beans to 4-qt. slow cooker.

2. Stir in 4 cups water and next six ingredients. Cover and cook on low setting for eight hours. Stir in fresh oregano and season with salt and pepper to taste.

SERVINGS: 8 | SOURCE: Little Rusted Ladle

COUSCOUS & BUCKWHEAT SALAD WITH OREGANO

This gorgeous salad is loaded with flavor and good for you as well. The oregano is present in both dried and fresh forms and works well with the earthy taste of turmeric, the salty feta, the sweet pomegranate, and the peppery arugula. The balsamic and avocado oil finish it off with that needed zing of acidity to make this salad one of the more complex salads you'll taste.

1¼ cup chicken or vegetable broth

½ tsp. turmeric

½ cup pearled couscous

2 Tbsp. avocado oil or extra virgin olive oil, divided

1½ cup water

¼ tsp. kosher salt

1 tsp. dried mexican oregano, crushed

½ cup buckwheat groats

1 cup baby arugula, washed

¼ cup fresh oregano leaves, loosely packed

¼ cup crumbled feta cheese

½ tsp. fresh ground black pepper

1 cup small broken pieces fresh cauliflower

½ cup pomegranate arils (seeds)

2 tsp. white balsamic vinegar

Salt to taste

1. FOR COUSCOUS, in a small saucepan, bring broth and turmeric to a boil. Reduce heat to low, stir in couscous. Cover and simmer for 10–12 minutes or until liquid is absorbed. Transfer cooked couscous to a small bowl, stir in half of the oil, cover, and let cool completely.

2. FOR BUCKWHEAT, in another small saucepan, bring water, salt, and dried oregano to a boil. Reduce heat to low, then add buckwheat. Cover and simmer for ten minutes or until liquid is absorbed. Transfer cooked buckwheat to a small bowl, stir in remaining oil, cover, and set aside to cool completely.

3. TO MAKE SALAD, in a large bowl, combine cooled couscous, buckwheat, and remaining ingredients. Toss gently to combine. Serve.

SERVINGS: 4 | SOURCE: Little Rusted Ladle

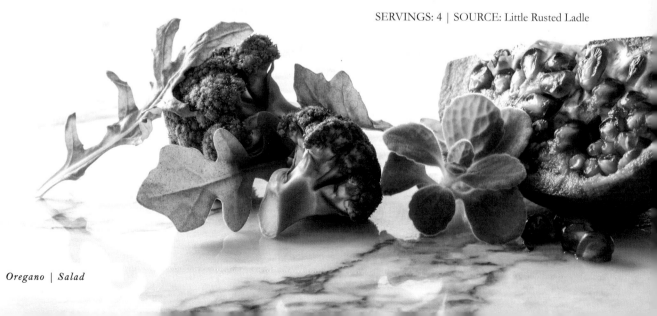

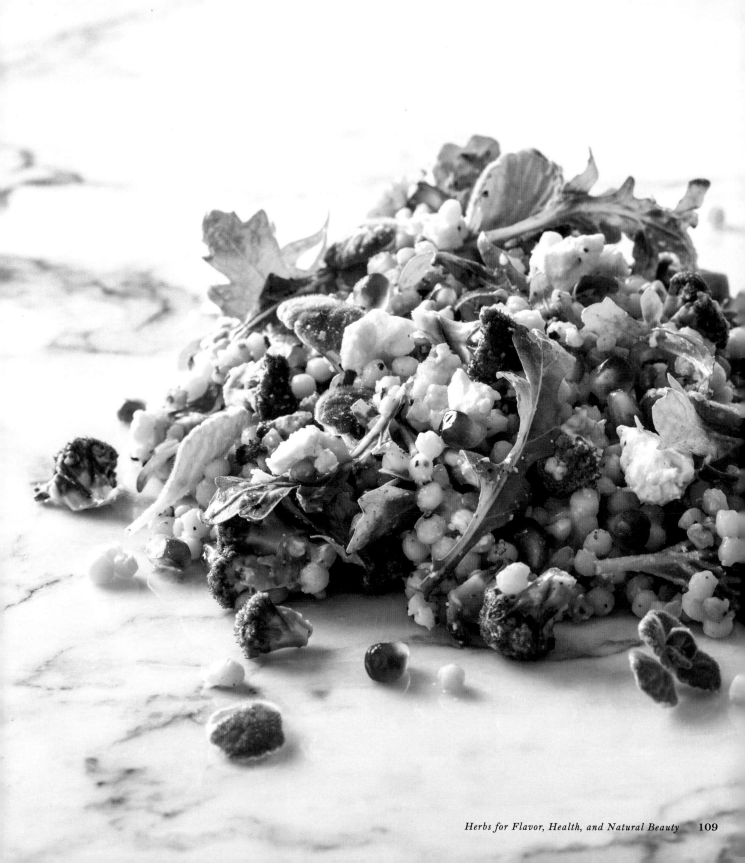

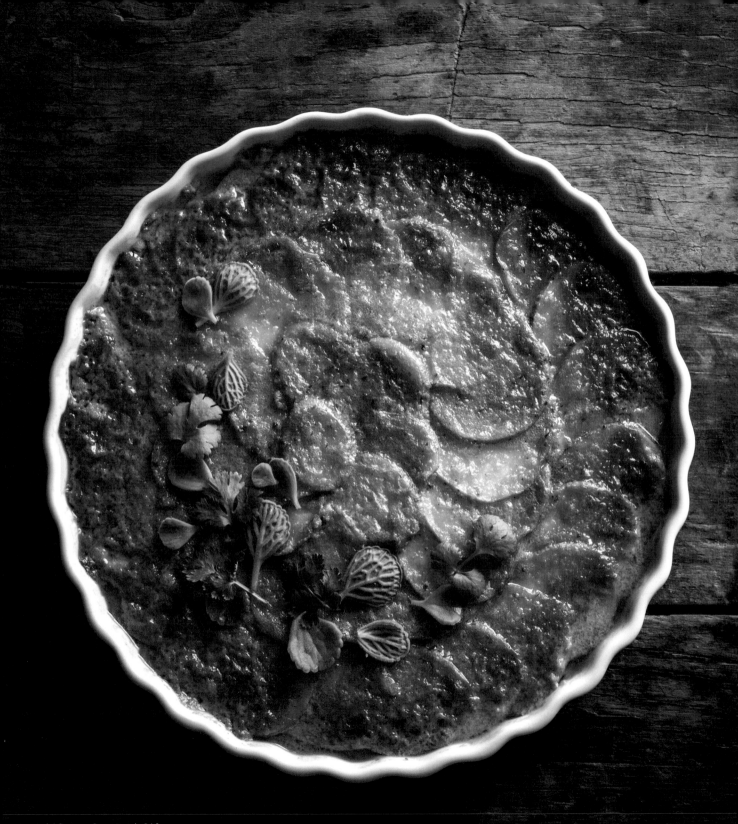

MEXICAN POTATOES WITH CUBAN OREGANO

This dish is a variation of the classic potatoes Anna. This time we use mexican cheeses, chipotle peppers, and fresh oregano and cilantro to give it that south-of-the-border feel. This dish can be made ahead and reheated in a 275 degree oven for 30 minutes. Cuban oregano works really well in this dish because it acts like a vegetable. The succulent nature of this slightly floral herb is a good contrast to the rich and cheesy potatoes.

¾ cup heavy cream, warmed

¼ cup chicken broth

3 Tbsp. unsalted butter, melted

¼ cup chipotle peppers in adobo sauce, finely chopped

1 tsp. seasoned salt

6 medium yukon gold or yellow potatoes, thinly sliced

2 cups shredded mexican blend cheese

½ cup diced anaheim peppers

¼ cup diced onion

½ cup cilantro leaves, loosely packed

½ cup cuban oregano leaves, loosely packed

1. Spray a 9-inch tart pan with nonstick spray. In a 2-cup glass-measuring cup, combine cream, broth, butter, chipotle peppers, and seasoned salt.

2. TO ASSEMBLE POTATOES, preheat oven to 350 degrees. Place potato slices overlapping in circles until the bottom of the tart pan is filled. Sprinkle ½ cup of cheese over potatoes, then sprinkle a couple of tablespoons of anaheim peppers and onions over cheese. Sprinkle about 2 tablespoons of herbs over peppers and onions. Pour ¼ cup of cream mixture over the top. Repeat process with remaining potatoes, cheese, vegetables, herbs, and liquid. Cover pan with foil and place on a sheet pan. Bake for 40 minutes. Remove foil and bake an additional 30 minutes or until top is golden brown and potatoes are tender. Remove from oven and let cool for about ten minutes. Top with additional oregano for garnish if desired and serve.

SERVINGS: 4 | SOURCE: Little Rusted Ladle

GREEK SHEPHERD'S PIE

The only word I can use to describe this dish is yummy. Don't be scared off by the list of ingredients. Each one has a purpose and adds another layer of flavor that when combined, produces a hearty, full-flavored dish that makes the original version pale in comparison.

1. FOR FILLING, combine oregano and next four ingredients in a re-sealable plastic bag. Add short ribs, seal bag, and move meat around in bag until evenly coated with seasoning. Add flour to bag and roll bag until flour coats meat. Preheat oven to 325 degrees. In a dutch oven, sear seasoned beef in oil on all sides until well browned (7–10 minutes). Transfer meat to a plate and set aside. Add remaining oil to dish and sauté onion and next seven ingredients over medium heat for about five minutes or until softened. Add broth, wine reduction, oregano, and bay leaf back to dutch oven. Add browned meat. Cover with lid and place on middle rack of oven. Cook for 90 minutes or until beef and vegetables are tender. Skim 2 Tbsp. of fat from top of beef mixture into a small bowl. Stir flour into fat. Add to cooked beef mixture and cook on stovetop for about 10 minutes or until mixture is thickened. Set dish aside to cool while making potatoes.

2. FOR POTATOES, place potatoes and parsnips in a large saucepan. Cover with water and bring to a boil. Reduce heat and cook on medium for 10–12 minutes or until potatoes are tender. Drain through a colander, then add back to saucepan. Mash potatoes with a potato masher. Add butter 2 tablespoons at a time until butter has melted into potatoes. Repeat with remaining butter until potatoes are creamy. Add cream and stir until light and creamy. Season to taste with salt and pepper.

3. TO ASSEMBLE DISH, spoon mashed potatoes into a re-sealable freezer bag. Remove as much air as possible. Cut a hole at the end of the bag with scissors leaving a 1-inch round hole. Pipe potatoes in circles over beef mixture. Drizzle with olive oil and paprika. Bake uncovered for 20–25 minutes or until mixture is hot and potatoes are lightly browned. Remove from oven and sprinkle with feta cheese and additional fresh oregano leaves if desired. Serve.

SERVINGS: 4 | SOURCE: Little Rusted Ladle

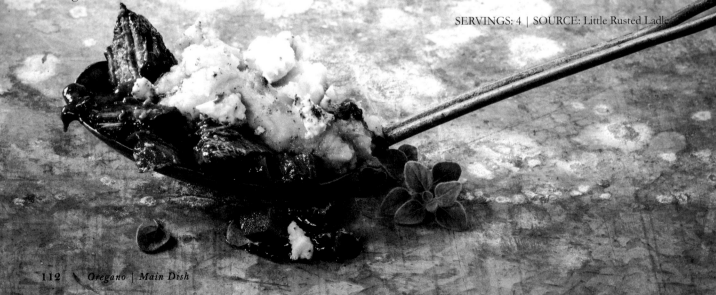

2 tsp. dried oregano

½ tsp. dried rosemary, crushed

½ tsp. dried thyme

½ tsp. black pepper

½ tsp. kosher salt

2 Tbsp. flour

1½ lbs. boneless beef short ribs, cut into pieces

3 Tbsp. EVOO, divided

1 cup onion, chopped

¾ cup celery, chopped

¾ cup carrots, peeled, sliced

½ cup red bell pepper, chopped

½ cup yellow bell pepper, chopped

½ cup green olives, sliced

4 cloves garlic, minced

½ cup sun-dried tomatoes, chopped

2 cups beef stock or broth

¼ cup fresh oregano leaves, loosely packed

1 ea. bay leaf

1½ lbs. small yellow potatoes, washed

2 large parsnips, peeled, chopped

6 Tbsp. unsalted butter

¼ cup heavy cream

Salt and pepper to taste

1 Tbsp. EVOO, optional

½ tsp. smoked paprika, optional

¼ cup feta cheese, crumbled

1 Tbsp. fresh oregano leaves, for garnish, optional

2 Tbsp. green olives, for garnish, optional

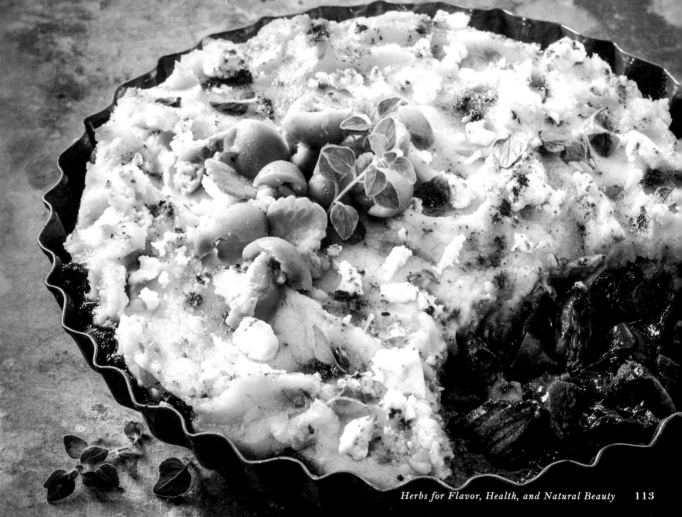

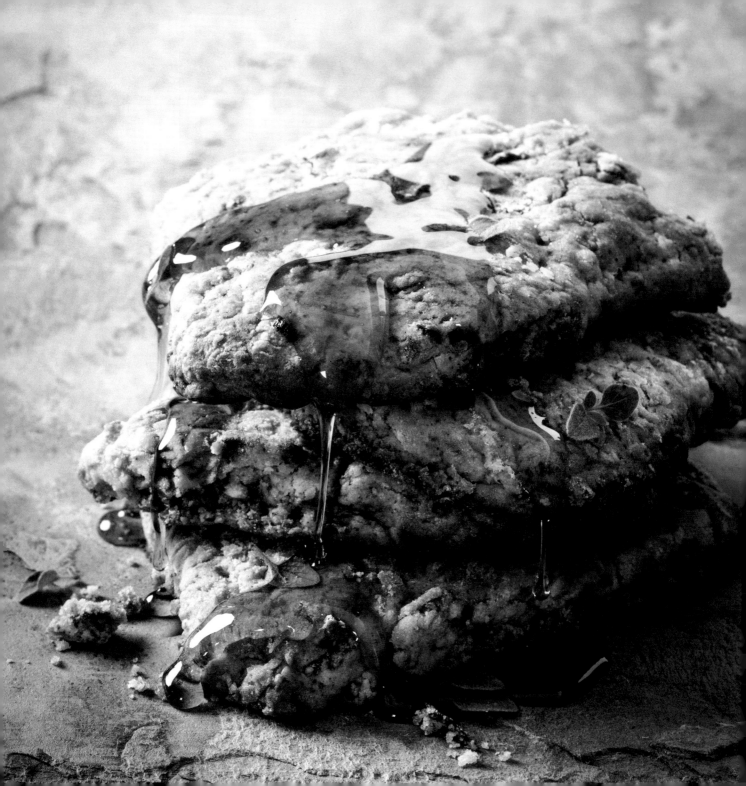

COCONUT GRAPE SCONES WITH OREGANO & HONEY

1½ cups unbleached flour

¼ cup sugar

1¼ tsp. baking powder

¼ tsp. baking soda

¼ tsp. salt

6 Tbsp. butter, chilled, cut into small pieces

½ cup buttermilk

½ cup freeze-dried grapes, finely ground

¼ cup unsweetened coconut, toasted

1 Tbsp. fresh oregano leaves

½ cup honey

These light and fluffy scones resemble biscuits more than they some of the hard and crumbly scones I've had in the past. Adding freeze-dried grape powder, toasted coconut, and fresh oregano is a very unique combination of sweet, floral, and tropical all folded into a fluffy biscuit. You could serve these scones topped with fresh fruit as well, but you may just find that the simple drizzle of honey is all you need. You can eliminate the freeze-dried grapes, but once you've tried powdered freeze-dried fruit in baked goods, you'll find yourself using it a lot. Only use fresh oregano with this recipe, as using dried will produce a scone that tastes a little too much like pizza.

1. IN A LARGE BOWL, combine flour and next four ingredients. Cut in butter with a fork or pastry blender until mixture resembles coarse meal.

2. Stir in buttermilk, ground grapes, coconut, and oregano leaves. Gently mix until dough forms. Form dough into a ball and transfer to a lightly floured flat surface. Press dough into a circle about 1-inch thick. Cut into eight wedges.

3. Place wedges on a sheet pan lined with parchment paper. Bake for 12–15 minutes or until lightly browned.

4. Cool on a wire rack. Serve with honey drizzled on top.

SERVINGS: 4 | SOURCE: Little Rusted Ladle

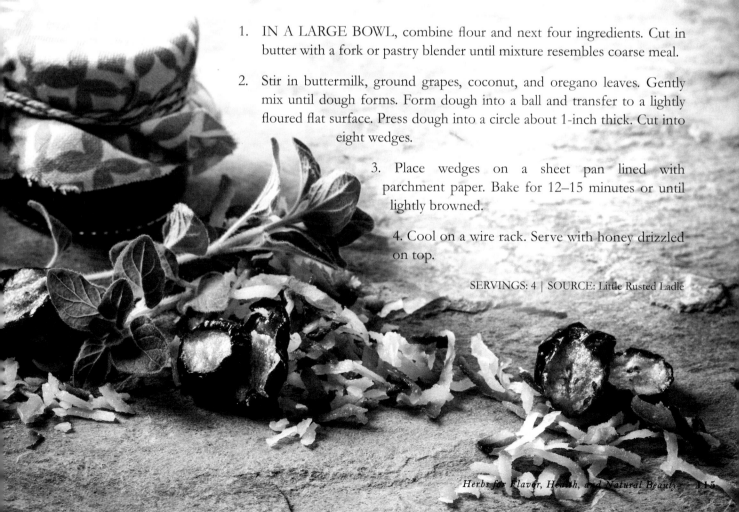

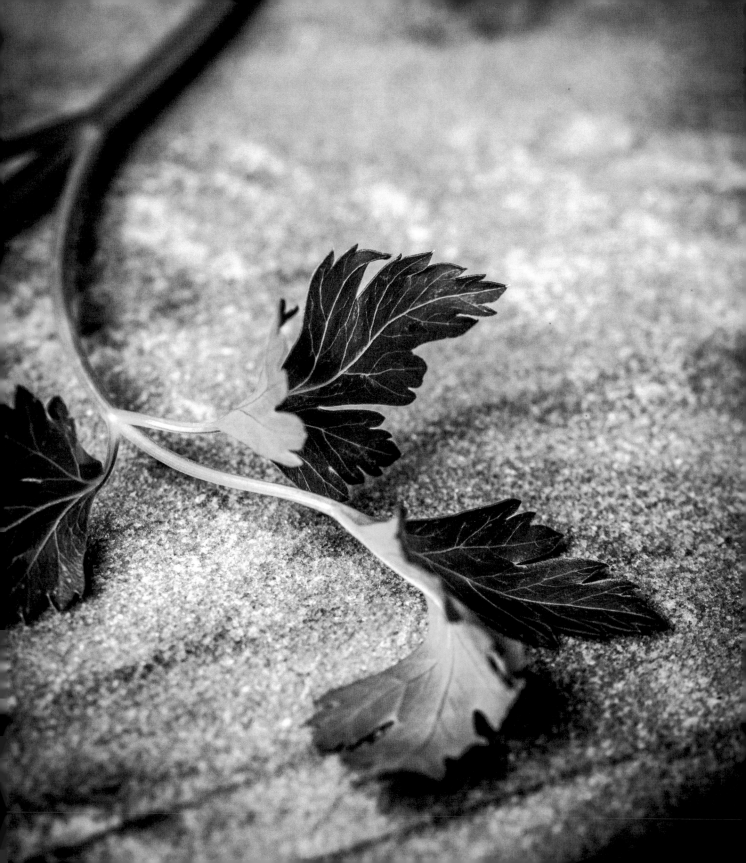

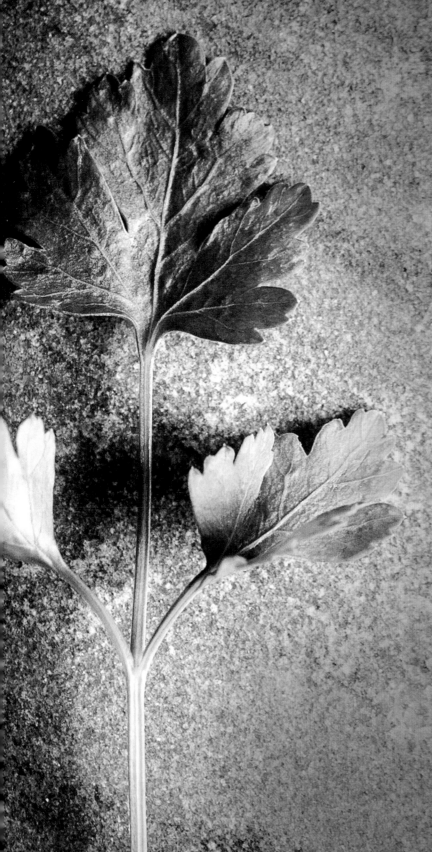

Chapter 9:
PARSLEY

*P*arsley has received a bad rap over the years. It has been poorly used as a token garnish by restaurant chefs and home cooks alike. However, parsley offers exceptional culinary opportunities, which have been enjoyed by chefs for hundreds of years. It also offers medicinal benefits as well. Did you know that ingesting parsley is an excellent way of removing heavy metals from the body and that the herb is found in many detoxification recipes? The versatility of parsley is incredible. From being one of the main ingredients in french cuisine's bouquet garni, to being used extensively in greek, italian and indian cuisines, parsley can do it all. It works well in both savory and sweet dishes as well as in beverages, dressings, soups, sauces, baked goods, and a myriad of other culinary creations. Parsley has a large taproot that tastes great in salads and soups. It's a cure for bad breath, it makes a wonderful addition to floral bouquets and wreaths, and it lasts a long time in harsh climates. Parsley deserves a lot of respect. Jena and I have put together a few uses for parsley that we hope shed some new light on this often abused and misunderstood herb.

FRESH HERB DIP

Sometimes you just want to dive into a bowl of dip with some pretzels or chips. The intense flavor of fresh parsley, basil, tarragon, and chives shine through with this tasty dip. Try it on chips, veggies, or pretzels. Feel free to substitute or add any other herbs you'd prefer including dill, lemon verbena, or cilantro. If blue cheese is not your preference, use goat cheese, cream cheese, or even cheddar, or omit the cheese all together.

¾ cup sour cream

¼ cup mayonnaise

¼ cup fresh parsley, chopped

¼ cup fresh herbs
(basil, chives, tarragon)

½ cup baby spinach

2 Tbsp. crumbled blue cheese

1 Tbsp. grated parmesan cheese

Salt and pepper to taste

1. Combine all ingredients in a food processor or blender. Blend until smooth. Serve.

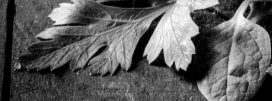

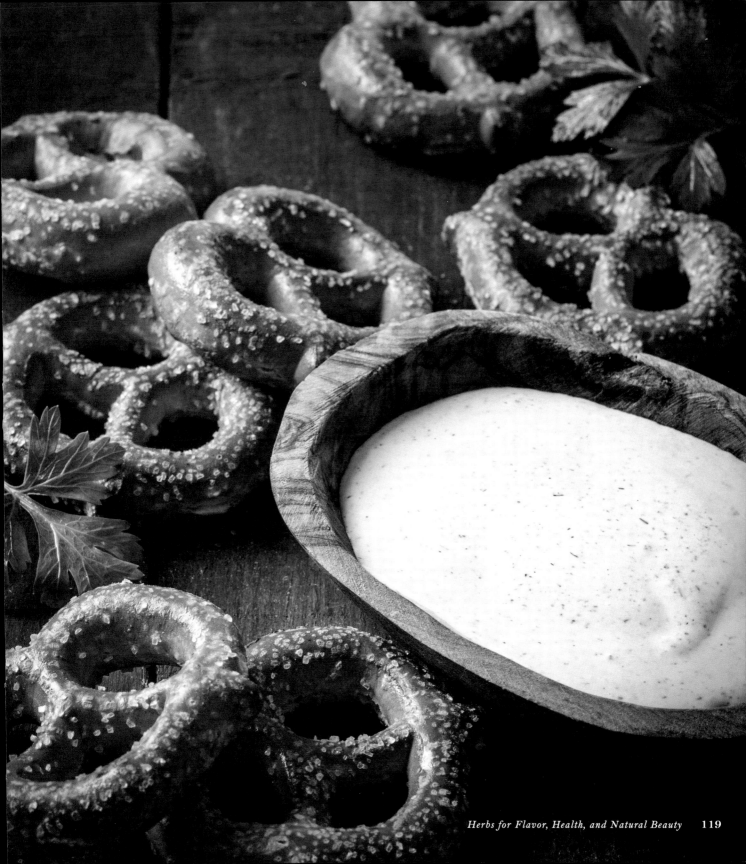

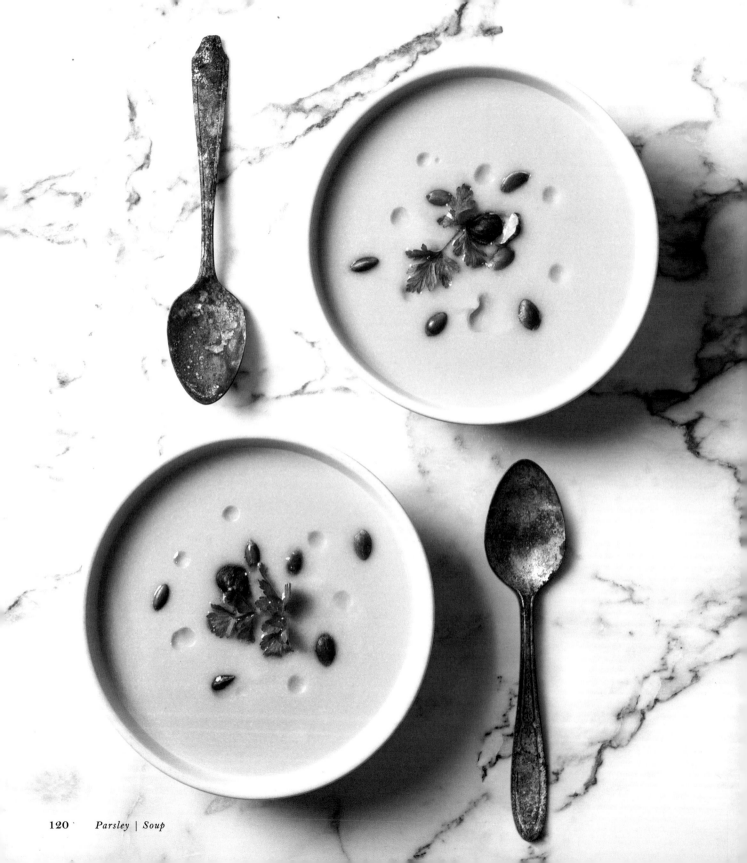

PARSNIP & PARSLEY ROOT BISQUE WITH WHITE TRUFFLE OIL

This easy-to-make sweet vegetable bisque gets a gourmet upgrade with the addition of white truffle oil and hazelnuts. It can also be made into a vegetarian soup by using vegetable broth in place of chicken broth.

4 cups (about 1 lb.) peeled and chopped parsnips or parsley root

2 cups whole milk

1 cup reduced-sodium chicken broth or vegetable broth

2 Tbsp. good-quality grated parmesan cheese

Salt and white pepper to taste

6–10 drops white truffle oil, optional

6–10 toasted hazelnuts

Reserved parsley sprigs (if using parsley root)

1. IN A LARGE SAUCEPAN, combine parsnips and/or parsley root, milk, and broth of choice. Simmer over medium-low heat for 15–20 minutes or until vegetables are very tender. Add mixture to a blender with parmesan cheese. Blend until smooth. Add salt and pepper to taste. Ladle into bowls. Sprinkle with white truffle oil, hazelnuts, and a parsley sprig.

SERVINGS: 4 | SOURCE: Little Rusted Ladle

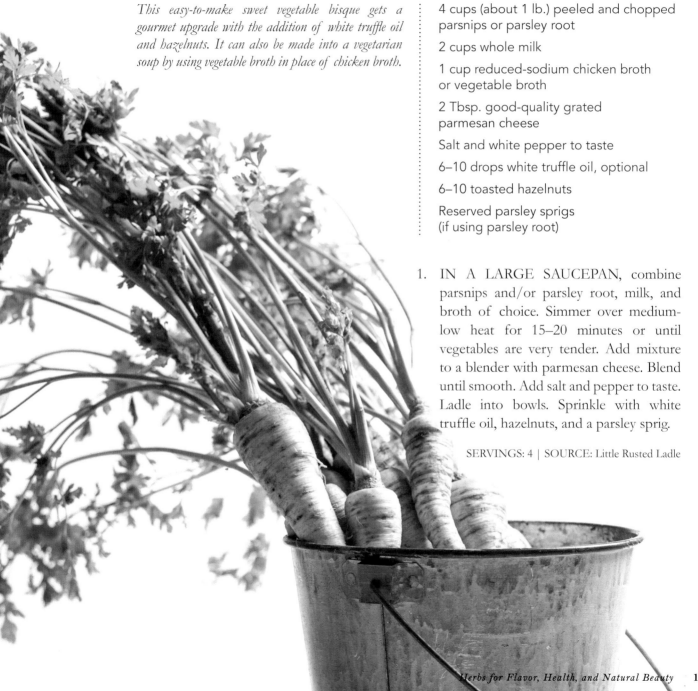

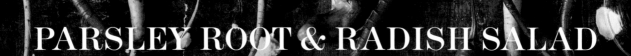

PARSLEY ROOT & RADISH SALAD

Parsley has the wonderful advantage of the whole plant being edible. Parsley root is related to parsnips, so you can use them interchangeably. They are less sweet and are slightly nutty. In this salad, they are used raw with wonderful thin slices of fresh radish and mild shishito peppers. The feta adds a nice salty balance and the garlic fried parsley leaves add a nice crunch at the end.

2 Tbsp. extra virgin olive oil	1 cup purple radishes	¼ cup crumbled feta cheese
2 garlic cloves, thinly sliced	1 cup watermelon or red radishes	½ tsp. kosher salt
½ cup fresh parsley leaves, loosely packed, washed and dried		1 Tbsp. apple cider or white wine vinegar
1 cup fresh parsley root, peeled	3 shishito peppers or bell peppers, thinly sliced	Fresh ground black pepper to taste
	½ cup chopped celery leaves	

1. **FOR GARLIC FRIED PARSLEY,** heat oil in a small saucepan. Add garlic and cook until lightly browned, about one minute. Remove quickly with a slotted spoon. Discard garlic. Add parsley leaves. Fry in remaining oil over medium heat until crisp, 30–45 seconds. Transfer fried parsley to a plate lined with paper towels. Set aside. Let remaining oil cool to add to salad.

2. **TO MAKE SALAD,** using a vegetable peeler, cut long strips of parsley root and radishes like you were peeling them. Transfer to a large bowl. Add cooled garlic oil, peppers, celery leaves, feta cheese, salt, and vinegar. Toss to coat. Transfer salad to plates and top with fried parsley leaves and pepper to taste. Serve.

SERVINGS: 4 | SOURCE: Little Rusted Ladle

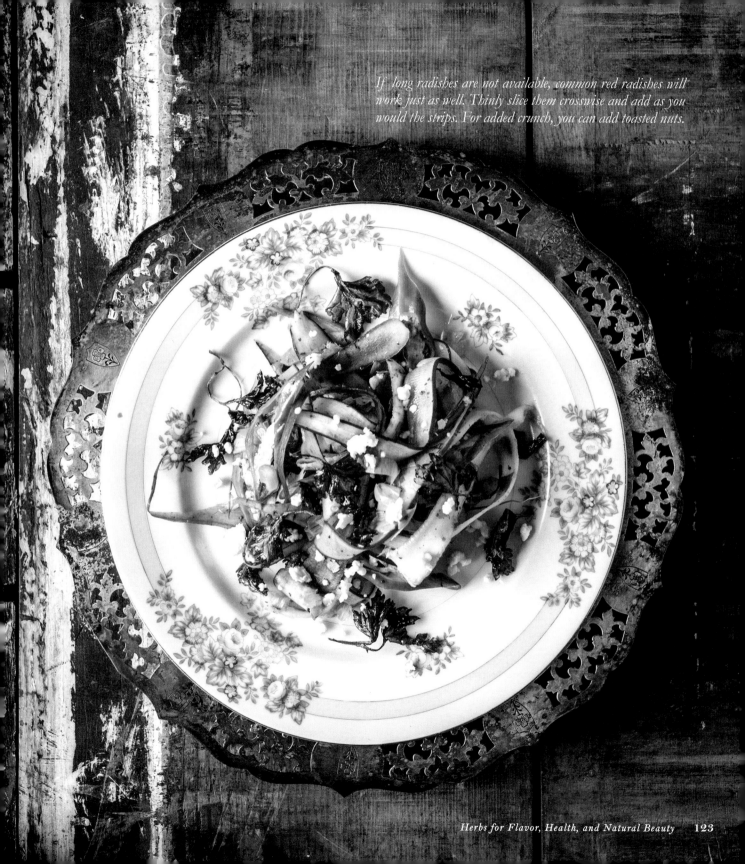

If long radishes are not available, common red radishes will work just as well. Thinly slice them crosswise and add as you would the strips. For added crunch, you can add toasted nuts.

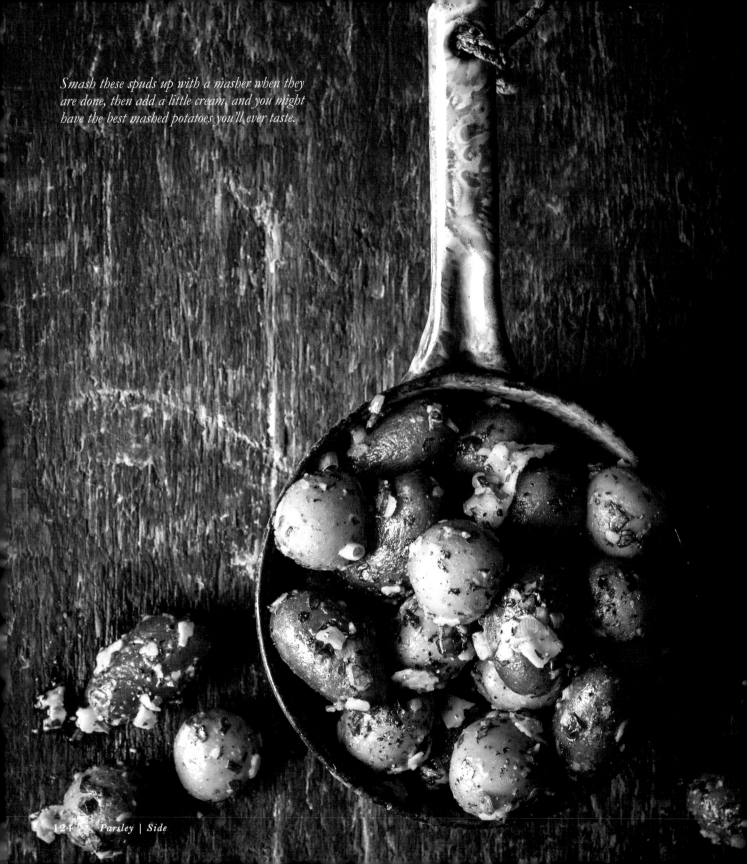

*Smash these spuds up with a masher when they
are done, then add a little cream, and you might
have the best mashed potatoes you'll ever taste.*

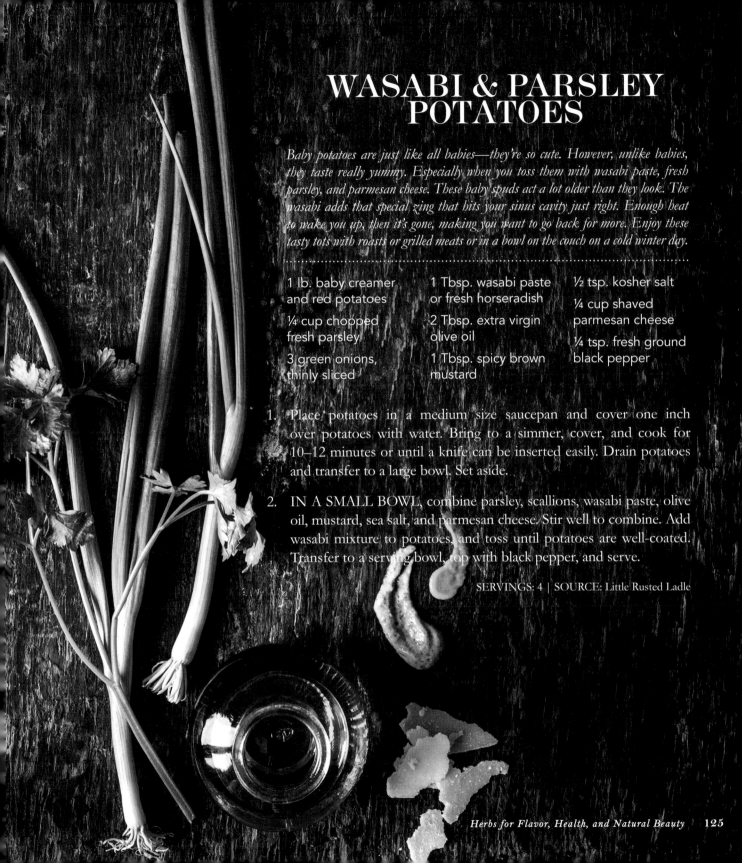

WASABI & PARSLEY POTATOES

Baby potatoes are just like all babies—they're so cute. However, unlike babies, they taste really yummy. Especially when you toss them with wasabi paste, fresh parsley, and parmesan cheese. These baby spuds act a lot older than they look. The wasabi adds that special zing that hits your sinus cavity just right. Enough heat to wake you up, then it's gone, making you want to go back for more. Enjoy these tasty tots with roasts or grilled meats or in a bowl on the couch on a cold winter day.

1 lb. baby creamer and red potatoes

¼ cup chopped fresh parsley

3 green onions, thinly sliced

1 Tbsp. wasabi paste or fresh horseradish

2 Tbsp. extra virgin olive oil

1 Tbsp. spicy brown mustard

½ tsp. kosher salt

¼ cup shaved parmesan cheese

¼ tsp. fresh ground black pepper

1. Place potatoes in a medium size saucepan and cover one inch over potatoes with water. Bring to a simmer, cover, and cook for 10–12 minutes or until a knife can be inserted easily. Drain potatoes and transfer to a large bowl. Set aside.

2. IN A SMALL BOWL, combine parsley, scallions, wasabi paste, olive oil, mustard, sea salt, and parmesan cheese. Stir well to combine. Add wasabi mixture to potatoes, and toss until potatoes are well-coated. Transfer to a serving bowl, top with black pepper, and serve.

SERVINGS: 4 | SOURCE: Little Rusted Ladle

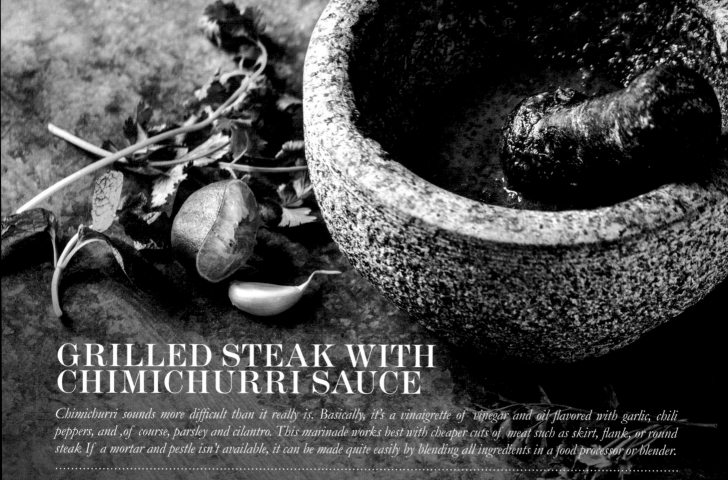

GRILLED STEAK WITH CHIMICHURRI SAUCE

Chimichurri sounds more difficult than it really is. Basically, it's a vinaigrette of vinegar and oil flavored with garlic, chili peppers, and ,of course, parsley and cilantro. This marinade works best with cheaper cuts of meat such as skirt, flank, or round steak If a mortar and pestle isn't available, it can be made quite easily by blending all ingredients in a food processor or blender.

1. FOR CHIMICHURRI SAUCE, using a mortar and pestle, smash garlic, parsley, cilantro, serrano pepper, red onion, and salt until a paste forms. Stir in red wine vinegar. While stirring, slowly add oil until all ingredients are incorporated. Set sauce aside.

2. FOR STEAK, add half of chimichurri sauce to a resealable plastic bag. Reserve remaining sauce for serving with the steak. Add steak to bag, seal top, and move steak around in sauce until well-coated. Refrigerate at least four hours.

3. Preheat grill on high if using a gas grill for about 15 minutes or until very hot. Transfer steak to a plate. Discard marinade. Let steak sit at room temperature for 15 minutes while grill is preheating. Grill steak over direct heat for about seven minutes per side or until medium rare. Transfer steak to a plate, sprinkle with salt and pepper, tent with foil, and let rest for 20 minutes. Slice steak and serve with reserved chimichurri sauce.

SERVINGS: 4 | SOURCE: Little Rusted Ladle

3 garlic cloves

½ cup chopped fresh parsley

¼ cup chopped fresh cilantro leaves

1 fresh serrano pepper, stem removed, cut into pieces

¼ cup chopped red onion

1 tsp. kosher salt

⅓ cup red wine vinegar

⅔ cup extra virgin olive oil

1½ lbs. beef round steak

Salt and pepper to taste

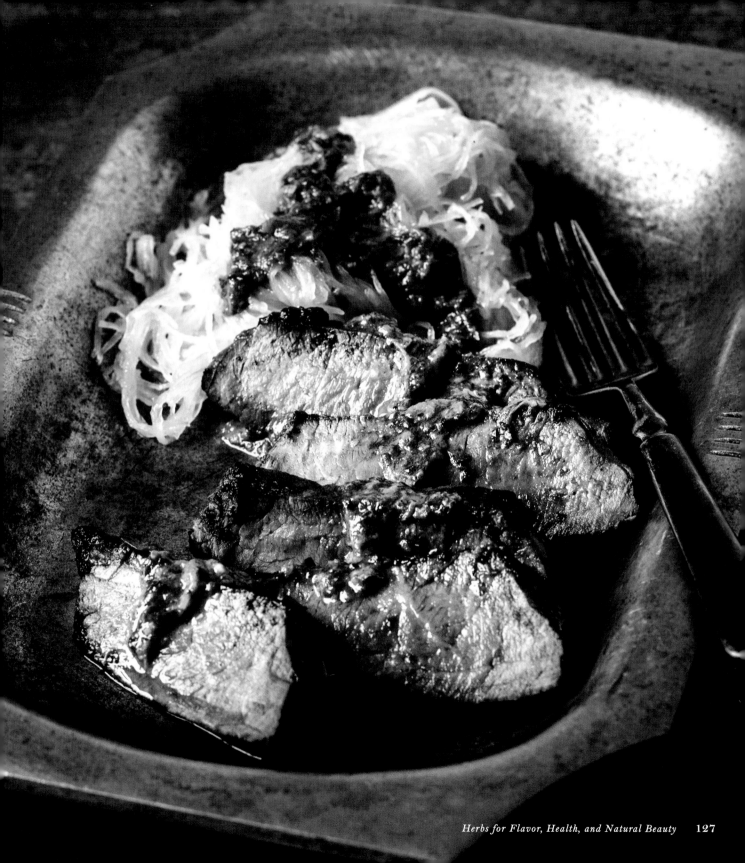

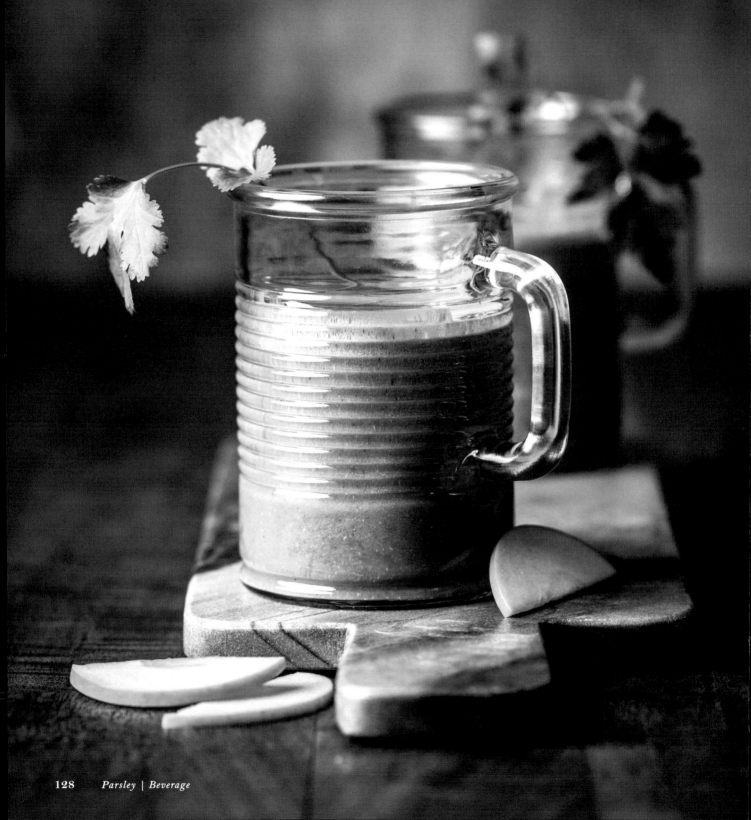

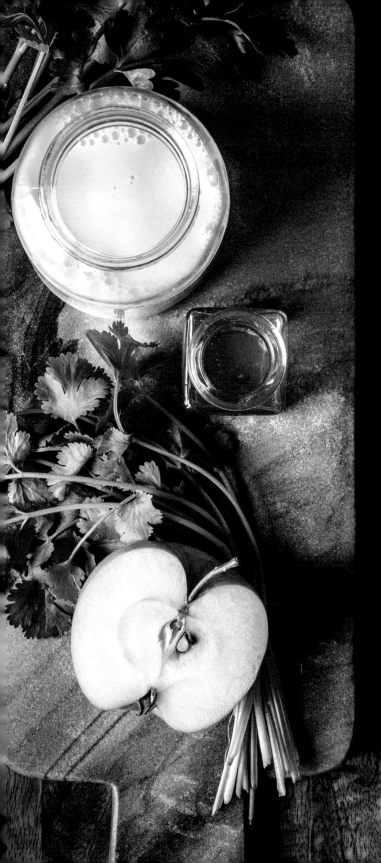

HEAVY METAL OATMEAL SMOOTHIE

Parsley and cilantro work hand in hand with this recipe. This cleansing powerhouse is a great way to help the body flush heavy metals from the body, while adding fiber and healthy fat. The apple, coconut milk, and honey give it a pleasantly sweet taste that makes this beverage taste better than it sounds. Your body will love you for it. This drink is best when consumed early in the morning on an empty stomach. If cilantro isn't your thing, double up on the parsley, or add some mint for more flavor.

½ cup leftover oatmeal, quinoa meal, or buckwheat meal

2 cup almond coconut milk or skim milk

1 cup coconut water

1 cup chopped green apple

½ cup fresh parsley, loosely packed

½ cup fresh cilantro, loosely packed

2 Tbsp. raw honey

6–8 ice cubes

1. Combine all ingredients in a blender. Blend on high until well-blended and smooth. Transfer to a glass and enjoy.

SERVINGS: 4 | SOURCE: Little Rusted Ladle

COCONUT ALMOND MILK & FRESH HERB POPSICLES

Sometimes the unexpected can be a wonderful surprise. Coconut almond milk has a great flavor on its own and is dairy free. Avocado has a natural creamy feel that goes great in frozen desserts. What's unexpected is that the parsley is a good addition. Adding honey as the sweetener, some lime juice for some acidity, and sliced fresh strawberries to the mix makes these popsicles good for you and good tasting too.

1 cup toasted coconut almond milk

1 cup chopped avocado

½ cup fresh parsley

2 Tbsp. honey

2 Tbsp. fresh lime juice

1 tsp. pure vanilla extract

1 pinch salt

½ cup sliced strawberries

1. Combine all ingredients except the strawberries in a blender. Blend until smooth. Divide mixture evenly into 5–6 oz. paper or plastic cups. Add strawberry slices. Place cups in an 8 x 8 pan. Cover each cup with a piece of plastic wrap. Pierce a hole in the middle of each covered cup. Place a stick in the hole and into the liquid. Freeze until firm. Remove from freezer. Remove popsicles by warming the sides of the cup with your hands until it releases. Serve immediately.

SERVINGS: 4 | SOURCE: Little Rusted Ladle

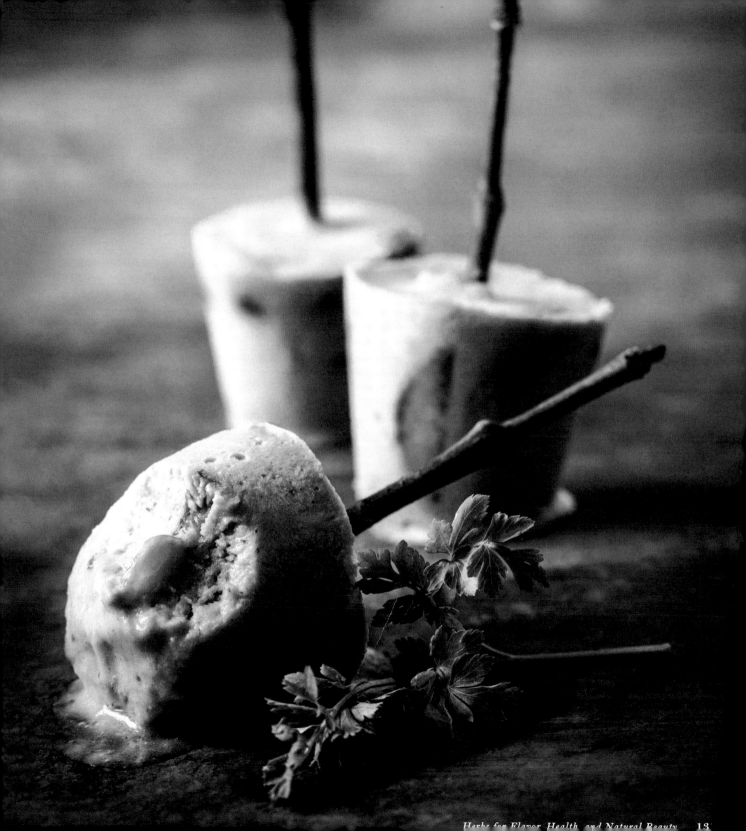

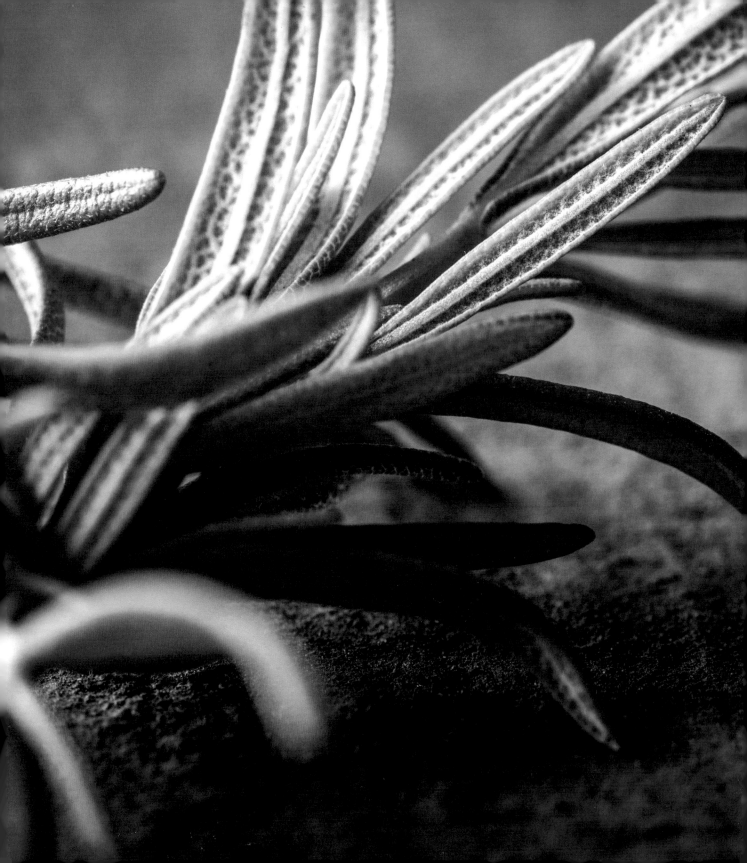

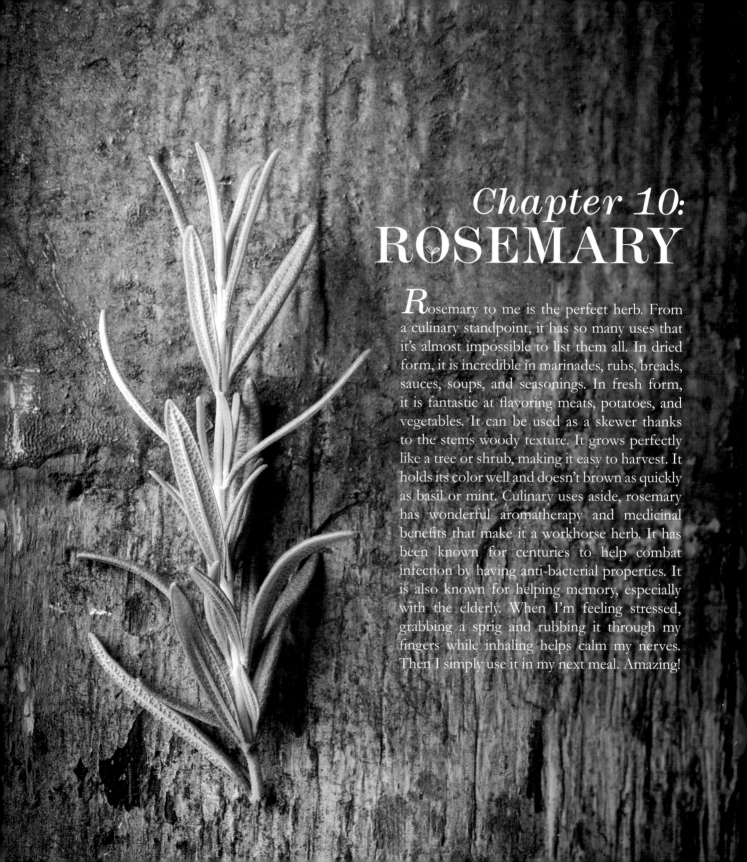

Chapter 10:
ROSEMARY

*R*osemary to me is the perfect herb. From a culinary standpoint, it has so many uses that it's almost impossible to list them all. In dried form, it is incredible in marinades, rubs, breads, sauces, soups, and seasonings. In fresh form, it is fantastic at flavoring meats, potatoes, and vegetables. It can be used as a skewer thanks to the stems woody texture. It grows perfectly like a tree or shrub, making it easy to harvest. It holds its color well and doesn't brown as quickly as basil or mint. Culinary uses aside, rosemary has wonderful aromatherapy and medicinal benefits that make it a workhorse herb. It has been known for centuries to help combat infection by having anti-bacterial properties. It is also known for helping memory, especially with the elderly. When I'm feeling stressed, grabbing a sprig and rubbing it through my fingers while inhaling helps calm my nerves. Then I simply use it in my next meal. Amazing!

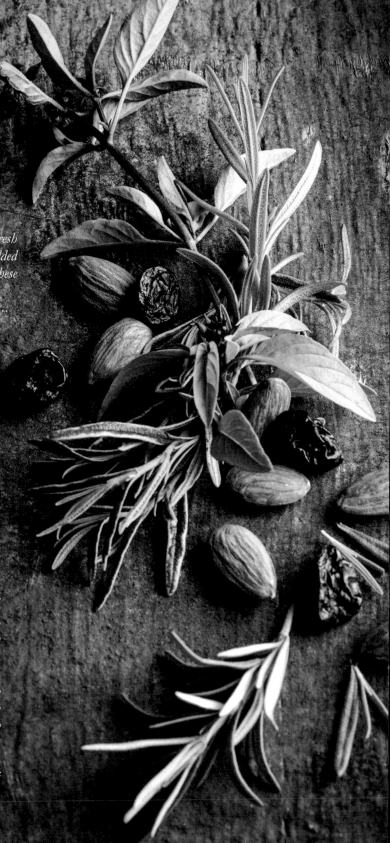

ROSEMARY ROASTED ALMONDS WITH DRIED CHERRIES

Almonds are a wonderful snack by themselves. Add fresh rosemary, basil, cinnamon, and dried cherries with the added flavor of smoked bacon and they become fantastic! Use these nuts by themselves or added to salads or snack mixes.

2 cups raw almonds

1 Tbsp. rendered bacon grease or butter

1 Tbsp. light brown sugar

2 Tbsp. finely chopped
fresh rosemary leaves

2 tsp. kosher salt

¼ tsp. ground cinnamon

½ tsp. fresh ground black pepper

2 tsp. finely chopped fresh basil leaves

1. Preheat oven to 325 degrees. In a medium bowl, combine almonds, bacon grease, and brown sugar. Toss to coat. Place almonds on a foil-lined sheet pan. Roast nuts for 15–20 minutes, stirring once after ten minutes, until lightly browned and sugar has melted onto nuts. Remove from oven and let cool completely.

2. IN A MEDIUM BOWL, combine rosemary, and next 4 ingredients. Transfer roasted nuts to bowl of rosemary cinnamon salt and toss to coat. Stir in dried cherries. Serve as a snack.

SERVINGS: 4 | SOURCE: Little Rusted Ladle

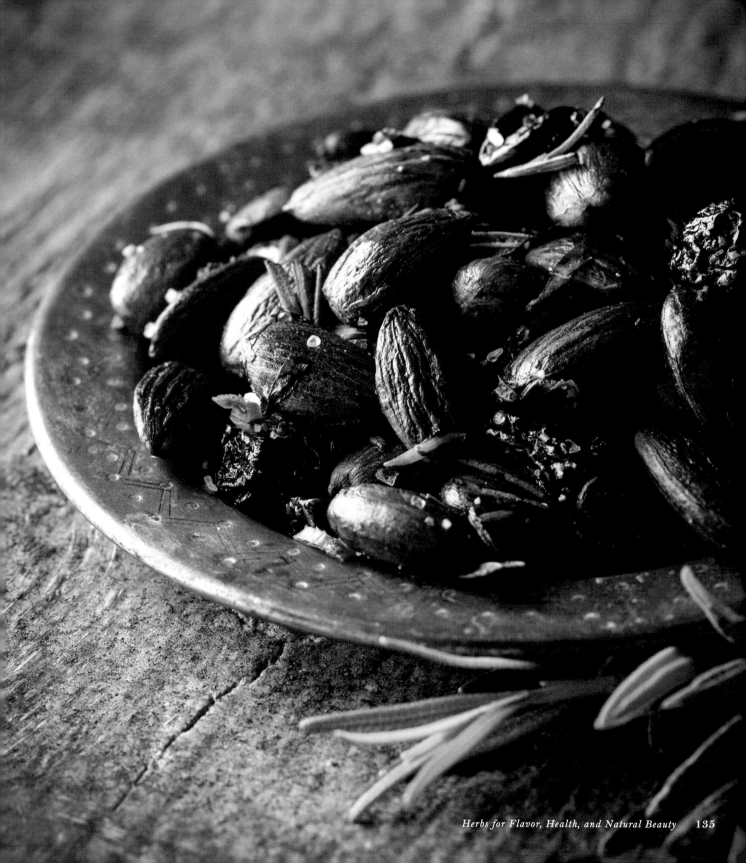

2 large sweet onions (3 cups), cut into strips

5 Tbsp. unsalted butter

4 cups beef broth

1 cup chicken broth

1 Tbsp. dried rosemary leaves, crushed

2 Tbsp. brown sugar

1 tsp. rosemary powder

4 dashes worcestershire sauce

2 tbsp. barbecue sauce

1 tsp. kosher salt

1 tsp. freshly ground black pepper

1 tsp. dried thyme

1 clove garlic, minced

1 ea. bay leaf

5 strips bacon, cut into ½-in. pieces

5 Tbsp. all-purpose flour

4 slices french bread, cubed

4 oz. cheddar cheese, shredded

2 oz. smoked swiss cheese, shredded

1 Tbsp. fresh rosemary leaves, finely chopped

5 Tbsp. unsalted butter, melted

2 cloves garlic, minced

1 Tbsp. fresh chives, chopped

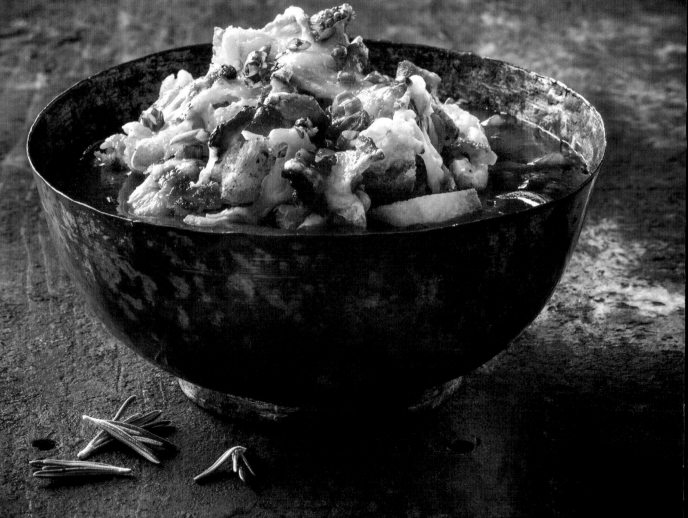

ROSEMARY ONION SOUP WITH CHEESY BACON CROUTONS

You know that classic french onion soup you see everywhere? Well, this isn't that soup. This is kind of a southern barbecue meets midwestern onion soup, and it's loaded with flavor. Instead of thyme, it's loaded with three kinds of rosemary. Instead of sherry, it's flavored with bourbon and a little barbecue sauce. Instead of gruyére cheese over a crouton, we top the soup with a cheesy bacon crouton that resembles pull apart bread. Enjoy!

1. FOR THE SOUP, cook onions in butter in a dutch over over medium heat for 10 minutes, stirring often. Reduce heat to low. Cook an additional 15 minutes or until golden brown. Add beef broth and next 11 ingredients. Simmer covered for 30 minutes. While soup is cooking, in a medium skillet, cook bacon over medium heat until browned. Transfer bacon with a slotted spoon to a plate lined with paper towels, reserving bacon grease. Make roux by stirring flour into bacon grease. Cook roux until deep golden brown, stirring often. Whisk roux into soup. Cook over medium heat until soup thickens. Keep hot until ready to serve.

2. FOR THE BACON CHEESE CROUTONS, preheat oven to 375 degrees. In a medium bowl, toss bread cubes with butter and garlic. Transfer to a foil-lined baking sheet. Bake in oven for eight minutes. Transfer bread cubes to a bowl. Add cheeses, rosemary, and cooked bacon. Toss to combine. Form into four mounds on the foil-lined baking sheet. Bake for 7–10 minutes or until cheese has melted into bread. Remove from oven and let cool for a minute while serving soup.

3. TO SERVE, ladle soup into bowls. Transfer bacon cheddar croutons on top of soup with spatula. Sprinkle with fresh chives. Serve.

SERVINGS: 4 | SOURCE: Little Rusted Ladle

ROASTED DOUBLE SQUASH SALAD WITH ROSEMARY DRESSING

This unconventional salad incorporates many fall flavors on one plate. The squash duo adds nice color, texture, and sweetness, while the wild rice adds a woodsy nuttiness. It has tartness from the cranberries, crunch from the seeds, and freshness from the lemon balm and parsley leaves. Of course, there is also the wonderful piney flavor that you get from two different sources of rosemary.

Don't eat the skin of the squash. It adds great color and texture, but that's about it.

1. FOR THE RICE, in a small saucepan, add wild rice, broth, and rosemary sprigs. Bring to a boil, then cover and reduce heat to low. Cook for 45–50 minutes or until wild rice is tender. Drain excess water and let cool. Remove rosemary sprigs and set aside.

2. FOR THE SQUASH, preheat oven to 375 degrees. Place acorn and butternut squash on a sheet pan. Drizzle 1 tablespoon of olive oil over squash and sprinkle with rosemary leaves, salt, and pepper. Roast for 15 minutes. In a small bowl, combine rosemary leaves, squash seeds, honey, and cranberry slices. Toss to coat. Add to pan with squash. Roast an additional 10–15 minutes or until squash is tender. Let cool to room temperature.

3. FOR THE DRESSING, in a small jar with a tight fitting lid, combine vinegar, remaining olive oil, rosemary, and maple syrup. Shake vigorously until thickened.

4. FOR THE SALAD, spoon some of the rice onto the platter. Place cooked squash over rice. Add parsley and lemon balm leaves, the remaining rice, and roasted squash seeds and cranberries. Season with salt and pepper to taste. Drizzle dressing over the top. Serve.

SERVINGS: 4 | SOURCE: Little Rusted Ladle

⅓ cup wild rice

1½ cups vegetable or chicken broth

2 sprigs fresh rosemary

1 delicata squash or ½ acorn squash, cut into slices, seeds reserved

1 butterkin squash or ½ butternut squash, cut into wedges, seeds reserved

3 Tbsp. light olive oil, divided

1 Tbsp. chopped fresh rosemary leaves

½ tsp. each salt and pepper

2 tsp. honey

¼ cup fresh cranberries, sliced

2 Tbsp. apple cider or white wine vinegar

2 Tbsp. avocado oil or extra virgin olive oil

2 Tbsp. maple syrup

1 Tbsp. italian parsley, chopped

4–5 fresh lemon balm leaves

4–5 fresh italian parsley leaves

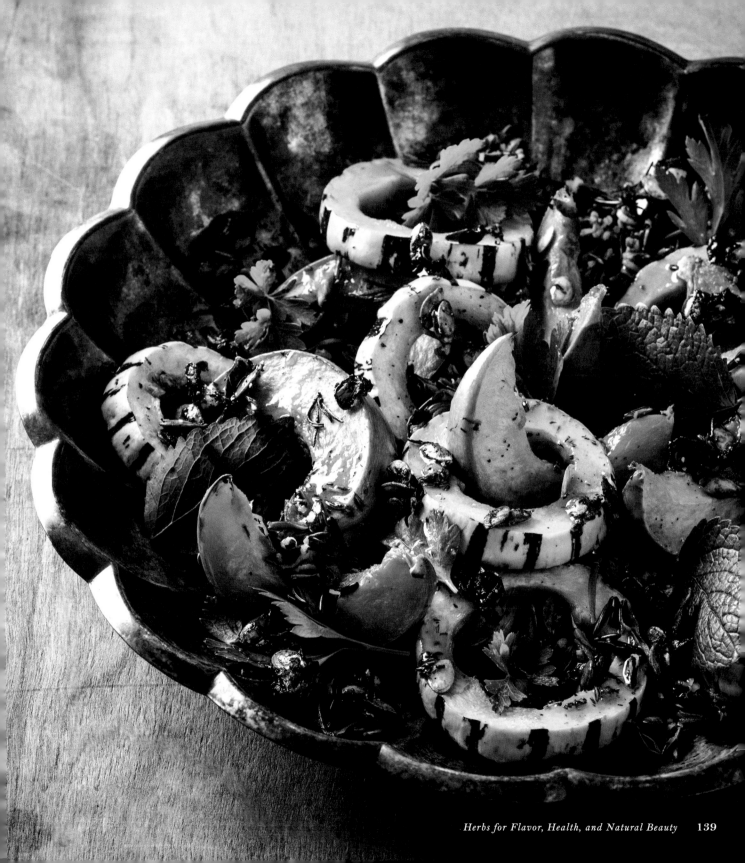

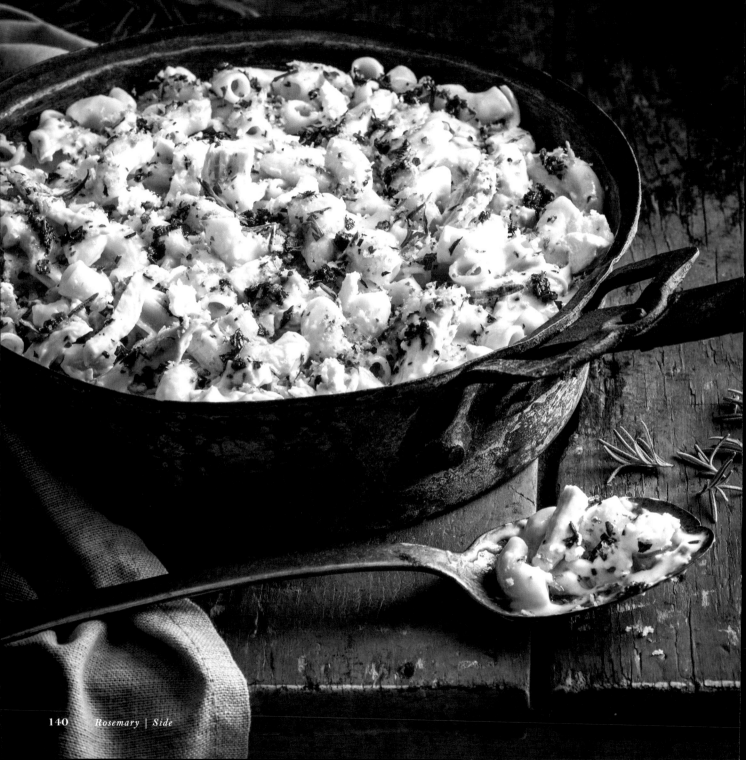

ROSEMARY CHICKEN MAC & CHEESE

Add more crumbled goat cheese on top if you desire a cheesier dish.

⅓ cup extra virgin olive oil

½ cup chopped fresh rosemary leaves, divided

2 cups chicken stock

2 cups water

2 cups heavy cream

3 cups large elbow macaroni

3 cups rotisserie chicken, cooked

4 oz. goat cheese, crumbled

Grape tomatoes

Salt and pepper to taste

½ cup panko bread crumbs

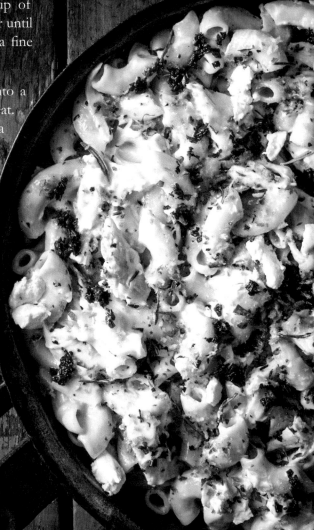

1. FOR ROSEMARY OIL, combine olive oil and ¼ cup of rosemary in a blender and blend on high for 1 minute or until rosemary is finely ground. Strain oil into a bowl with a fine strainer. Set rosemary oil aside.

2. FOR PASTA, pour chicken stock, water, and cream into a large dutch oven or saucepan. Bring to a boil over high heat. Reduce heat to medium, then add macaroni. Stir with a rubber spatula to prevent pasta from sticking. Cook for 8–10 minutes, stirring occasionally until pasta is al dente and liquid has thickened. Fold in chicken, goat cheese, and remaining rosemary. Cook 2–3 minutes longer or until goat cheese has melted into sauce. Add grape tomatoes. Cook for an additional 1–2 minutes. Season to taste with salt and pepper. Turn off heat and let rest for 2–3 minutes.

3. FOR CRUMB TOPPING, in a small skillet over medium heat, toast panko crumbs with 2 teaspoons of reserved rosemary oil for 2–3 minutes until crumbs are golden brown, stirring often. Remove from heat and let cool while you dish up mac and cheese.

4. TO SERVE, spoon macaroni mixture into shallow bowls or large mugs. Spoon 1–2 teaspoons of reserved rosemary oil over macaroni. Top with toasted rosemary crumbs. Serve.

SERVINGS: 4 | SOURCE: Little Rusted Ladle

ROSEMARY TURKEY PATTY MELTS

1⅓ lbs. lean ground turkey

½ cup fresh rosemary leaves, loosely packed, finely chopped

2 Tbsp. fresh sage leaves, finely chopped

1 Tbsp. fresh parsley leaves, finely chopped

1 Tbsp. fresh basil leaves, finely chopped

1 garlic clove, minced

1 tsp. kosher salt

1 Tbsp. worcestershire sauce

2 Tbsp. peach preserves, melted

¼ cup mayonaise

1 Tbsp. unsalted butter

1 cup thinly sliced onion

1 tsp. dried rosemary, crushed

4 slices havarti cheese, optional

8 slices brioche bread

1 cup baby spinach

1. Preheat grill. In a medium bowl, mix together turkey and next seven ingredients. Form into four equal patties and set aside. In a small bowl combine peach preserves and mayonnaise. Set aside.

2. IN A LARGE NONSTICK SKILLET, melt butter over medium heat. Add onion and dried rosemary. Sauté for 5–7 minutes, stirring often, or until onions begin to brown. Reduce heat to low, cook an additional 10 more minutes or until golden brown. Transfer onions to a small dish and set aside.

3. Grill reserved burger patties for five minutes on each side or until completely cooked on the inside. Place cheese slices on burgers, then transfer to a plate and tent with foil while grilling bread.

4. In the same pan that you sautéed the onions, preheat pan to medium-low heat. Brush one side of each bread slice with reserved peach mayo. Grill slices mayo-side down for 2–3 minutes or until golden brown. Top one piece of grilled bread on a plate. Top with some spinach leaves, a cooked burger, and grilled onions. Spoon a couple teaspoons of remaining mayo on top and finish with remaining slice of grilled bread. Repeat with remaining bread, spinach, burgers, onions, and mayo. Enjoy.

SERVINGS: 4 | SOURCE: Little Rusted Ladle

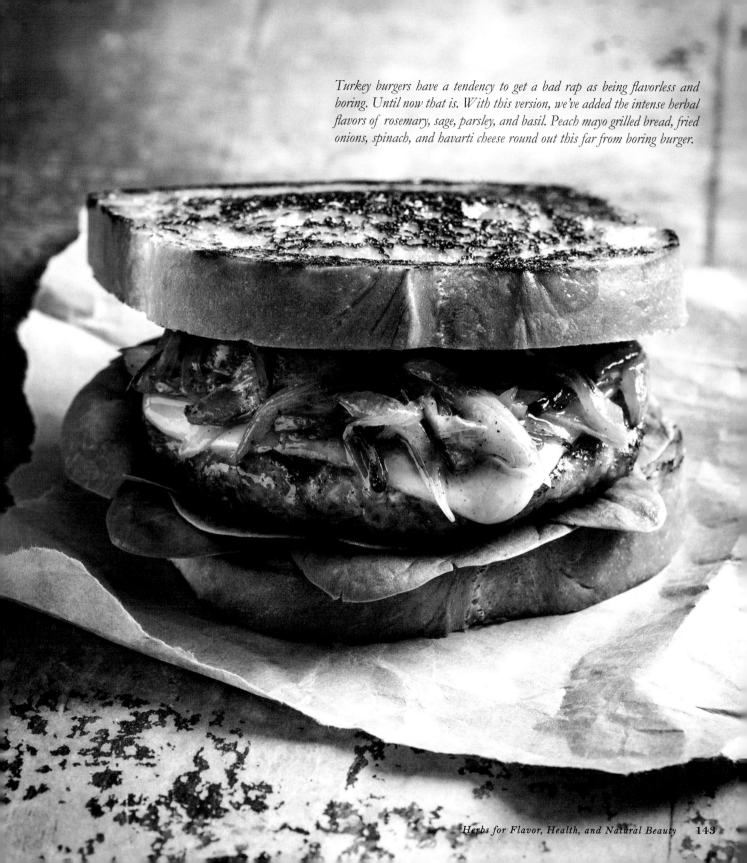

Turkey burgers have a tendency to get a bad rap as being flavorless and boring. Until now that is. With this version, we've added the intense herbal flavors of rosemary, sage, parsley, and basil. Peach mayo grilled bread, fried onions, spinach, and havarti cheese round out this far from boring burger.

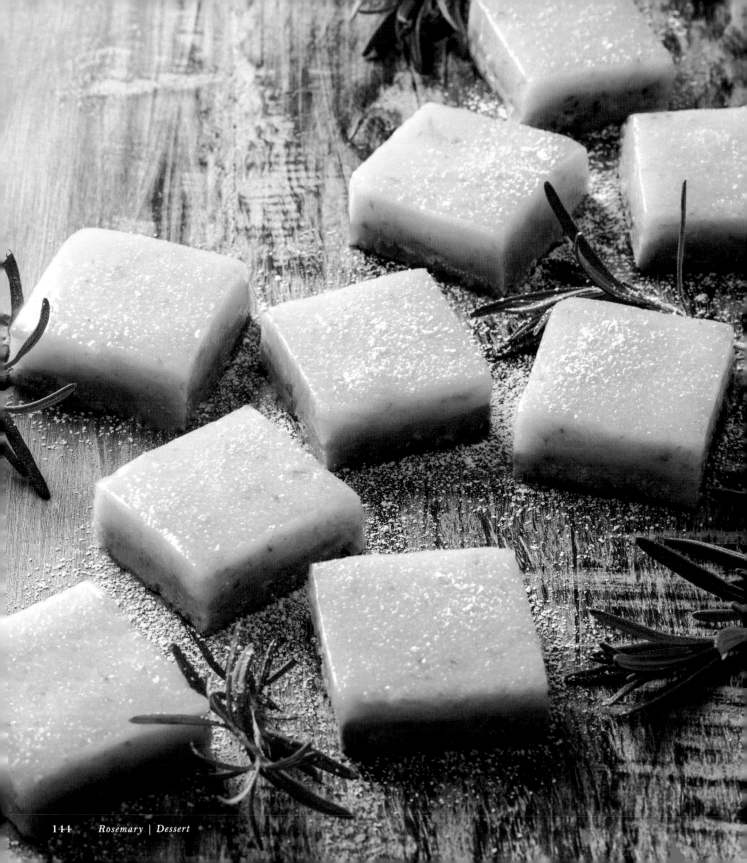

TRIPLE CITRUS BARS WITH ROSEMARY

The only thing better than lemon bars is lemon-lime-orange bars. Add a rosemary-infused shortbread crust, and you've got a dessert bar that will make people asking for the recipe every time they taste one. The olive oil adds a nice floral note that takes it to the top.

1 cup flour

10 Tbsp. unsalted butter, cut into cubes

¼ cup sugar

3 Tbsp. powdered sugar

1 pinch salt

1 Tbsp. finely chopped fresh rosemary leaves

1 tsp. zest each from lemon, lime, and orange

3 lemons

2 limes

1 orange

1½ cups sugar

2 large eggs, beaten

3 large egg yolks

2 tsp. cornstarch

¼ tsp. kosher salt

1 sprig fresh rosemary, optional

4 Tbsp. unsalted butter

¼ cup extra virgin olive oil

Powdered sugar, for garnish

Rosemary sprigs, for garnish, optional

1. FOR CRUST, preheat oven to 325 degrees. Line an 8 x 8 baking pan with parchment paper. In a food processor, combine flour and next five ingredients. Pulse 2–3 times. Add butter and pulse until crumbly dough forms. Press dough into the prepared pan and bake for 30–35 minutes or until light brown. While shortbread is baking, prepare citrus filling.

2. FOR TRIPLE CITRUS FILLING, grate 1 teaspoon each from peels of 1 lemon, 1 lime, and 1 orange. Transfer zest to a small dish and set aside. Juice lemons, limes, and orange to equal ¾ cup of juice. In a small saucepan, whisk together juice, sugar, eggs, egg yolk, cornstarch, salt, and rosemary sprig. Whisk mixture over medium-low heat for 3–5 minutes. When mixture starts to thicken, remove rosemary sprig. Continue whisking until mixture has thickened. Remove from heat and strain into a bowl. Whisk in butter, olive oil and reserved zest.

3. When crust is done baking, remove from oven and slowly pour triple citrus curd over crust. Return pan to oven and bake for 12–15 minutes or until topping is just set. Cool to room temperature, then refrigerate until cold. Cut into bars and dust with powdered sugar and top with a sprig of rosemary if desired. Enjoy.

SERVINGS: 8
SOURCE: Little Rusted Ladle

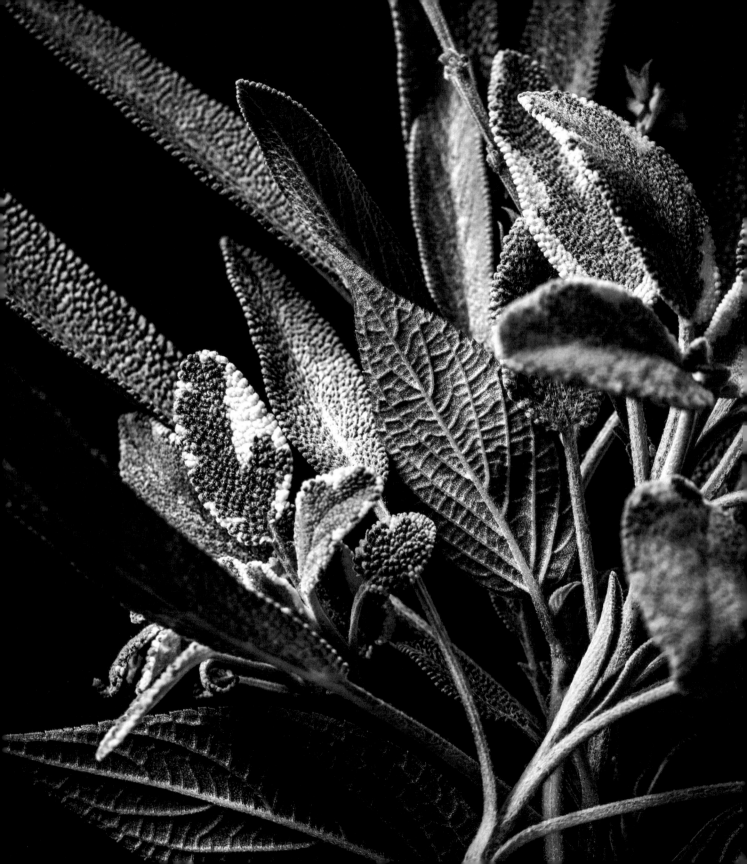

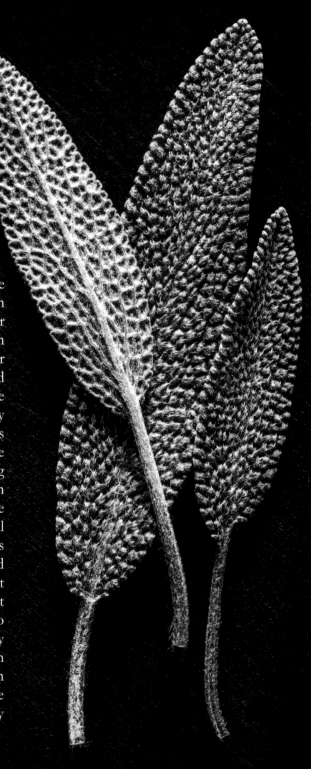

Chapter 11:
SAGE

*I*s there an herb that says "holiday season" more than the scent of sage wafting through the air on Thanksgiving Day? Sage may be known as the major herb used in stuffing and to season the turkey in late November, but there are a lot more uses for this storied herb than the Thanksgiving feast. Did you know that sage is known to be helpful in the treatment of dozens of ailments and everyday concerns? For example, for hundreds of years, this herb has been linked to helping prevent cognitive decline and actually helps give the mind a feeling of well-being. Its antibacterial properties have been used to kill harmful organisms in meats since the age of the Romans. Sage also has many nutritional benefits such as its above-average levels of vitamins K, B, C, E, fiber, riboflavin, calcium, iron, and folic acid, among others. It is also used to treat muscle aches and rheumatism. Did I mention that it is delicious used in cooking too? Sage added to meats, grains, soups, and vegetables turn normally boring dishes into ones that get handed down from generation to generation. So this November, when the turkey comes out of the oven smelling like sage and you breathe in deep, know that you are actually doing your body good. Enjoy.

FRIED SAGE BOUQUETS

If ever there was a recipe that celebrated the pure flavor of sage, it would be this one. The sage leaves are perfect for battering and frying. The leaves stay crisp for a long time. It's a great way to get rid of some extra sage in the fall, and your guests will love them. Feel free to experiment with different herbs like basil, lemon balm, tarragon, parsley, and greek oregano. When you're done frying, strain the oil and keep it for when you're cooking with turkey or chicken. The oil really picks up the flavor of the sage. Brush it on bread for a wonderful sage flavor.

½ cup rice flour

½ tsp. salt

1 large egg yolks

¼ cup ice water

6 large sage sprigs, 5–8 leaves per sprig, cleaned and dried

Parmesan cheese, optional

1. FOR THE BATTER, whisk rice flour, salt, egg yolk, and ice water in a medium size bowl until smooth. Refrigerate until ready to fry.

2. TO FRY THE BOUQUETS, remove batter from refrigerator and whisk until smooth again. Holding one of the sage sprigs by the stem, dip the sprigs leaf-first into the batter, turning it so that all the leaves are coated with batter. Quickly transfer to the pot of hot oil. Fry for 30 seconds, then turn over with a pair of small tongs. Fry an additional 30–45 seconds or until lightly browned and crispy. Remove fried sage with tongs, and transfer to a plane lined with paper towels. Repeat with remaining sage sprigs. Serve immediately.

SERVINGS: 4 | SOURCE: Little Rusted Ladle

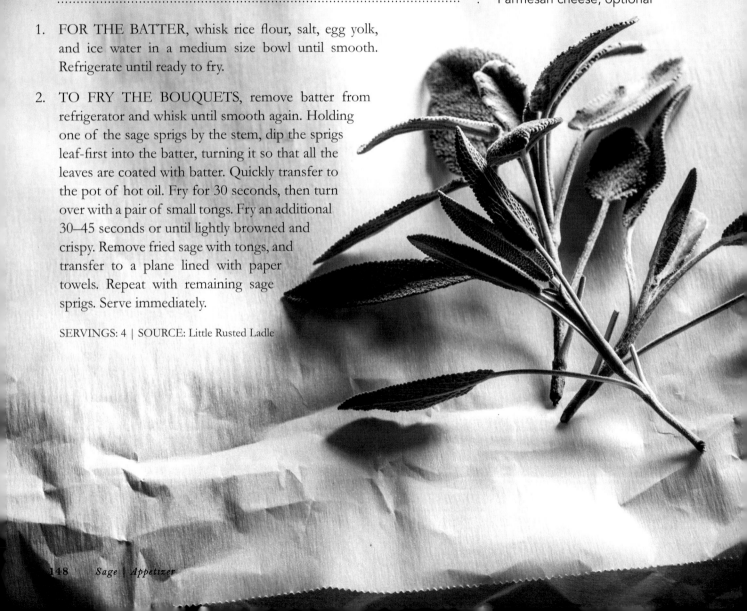

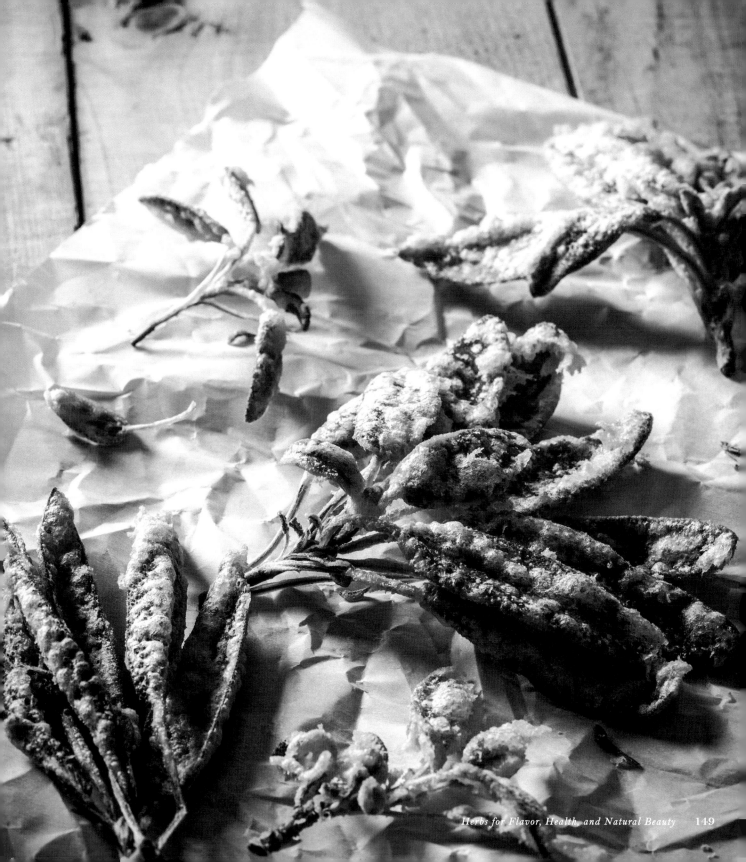

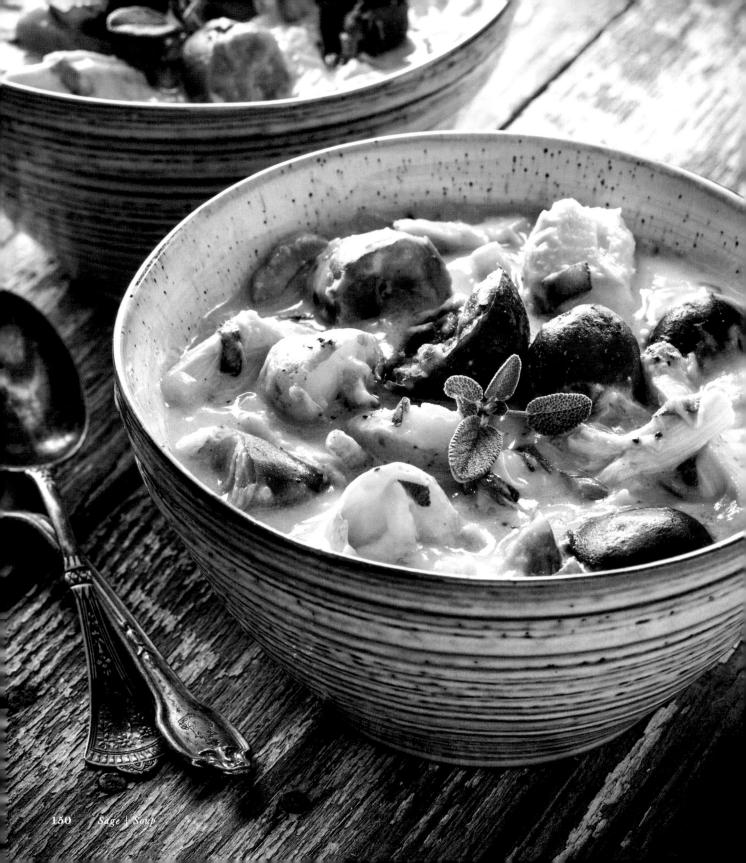

SAGE ROASTED CHICKEN CHOWDER

Nothing warms the soul like a big bowl of potato soup in the fall. Baby potatoes are surrounded by a rich and creamy soup base with the robust flavor of fresh sage. Pulled rotisserie chicken is added to make this hearty soup the perfect medicine for a cold and rainy day.

2 cups chicken broth	1 cup chopped celery
3 cups milk	5 Tbsp. flour
2 cups baby potatoes (red, yellow, or blue)	½ cup chopped fresh sage leaves
5 Tbsp. unsalted butter, divided	1½ cup pulled cooked rotisserie chicken
1 cup diced onion	1 tsp. kosher salt

1. IN A MEDIUM SAUCEPAN, combine chicken broth and milk. Add potatoes. Liquid should cover potatoes. Bring to a simmer over medium-low heat. Cover and cook for 12–17 minutes or until potatoes break in half when pierced with a fork. Transfer potatoes to a bowl with a slotted spoon, leaving broth mixture in the saucepan. Add 1 tablespoon of butter to the bowl. Stir until butter is melted. Cover potatoes and set aside. Keep broth mixture warm until ready to add roux.

2. While potatoes are cooking, in a medium skillet, melt 4 tablespoons butter over medium heat. Add onions and celery. Sauté mixture for 3–5 minutes or until softened. Add flour and sage. Stir until roux forms. Cook for 2–3 minutes or until roux is light brown in color.

3. Stir cooked roux into warm broth. Increase temperature to medium. Cook for 10–15 minutes or until thickened and hot. Stir in chicken and half of potatoes. Serve with warm buttered potatoes over the top. Garnish with fresh sage.

SERVINGS: 4 | SOURCE: Little Rusted Ladle

APPLE SAGE SALAD WITH MUSTARD-GLAZED WALNUTS & TRUFFLE HONEY

This sage salad recipe features fresh apples, mustard glazed walnuts, honey, truffle oil, and, of course, fresh sage. Each ingredient adds another layer of flavor. Using a spiral cutter, which is currently in trend, creates a pasta-like appearance, which gives the apples volume. If you don't have a spiral cutter, simply cut the apples into strips or thinly slice them. Drizzle the honey just before serving to prevent the apples from losing their crunchy texture.

3 large granny smith apples, peeled

2 Tbsp. lemon juice

2 cups water

¼ cup chopped walnuts

2 Tbsp. honey mustard

½ Tbsp. unsalted butter

¼ tsp. kosher salt

2 tsp. light olive oil

¼ cup fresh sage leaves, chopped

Fresh ground black pepper

4 tsp. honey, warmed

4–5 drops white truffle oil, optional

Small sage leaves, for garnish

1. Spiral cut apples using a spiral cutter, or cut apples into matchsticks. In a large bowl, combine lemon juice and water. Soak apples in lemon water for ten minutes while preparing nuts.

2. IN A SMALL SKILLET OVER MEDIUM HEAT, toast nuts until lightly browned, stirring often. Add honey mustard and butter. Toss to coat nuts. Cook for 1–2 minutes or until nuts are well-glazed. Transfer nuts to plate lined with parchment paper and cool completely. Set aside.

3. Drain apples from lemon juice completely. In a large bowl, gently toss apples, sage, and pepper. Drizzle with honey and truffle oil. Sprinkle nuts on top. Serve with small sage leaves as a garnish.

SERVINGS: 4 | SOURCE: Little Rusted Ladle

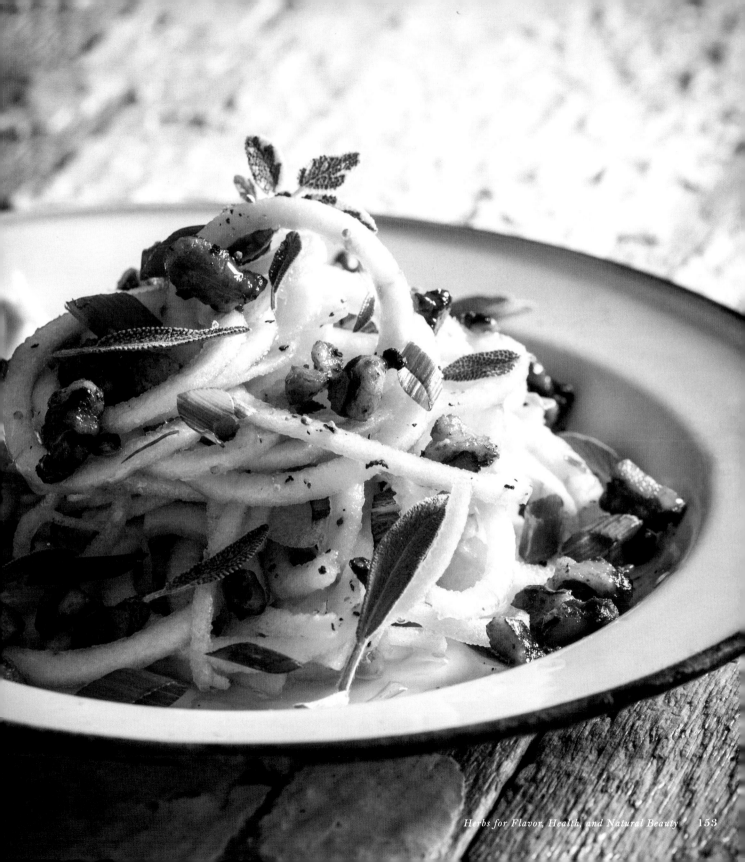

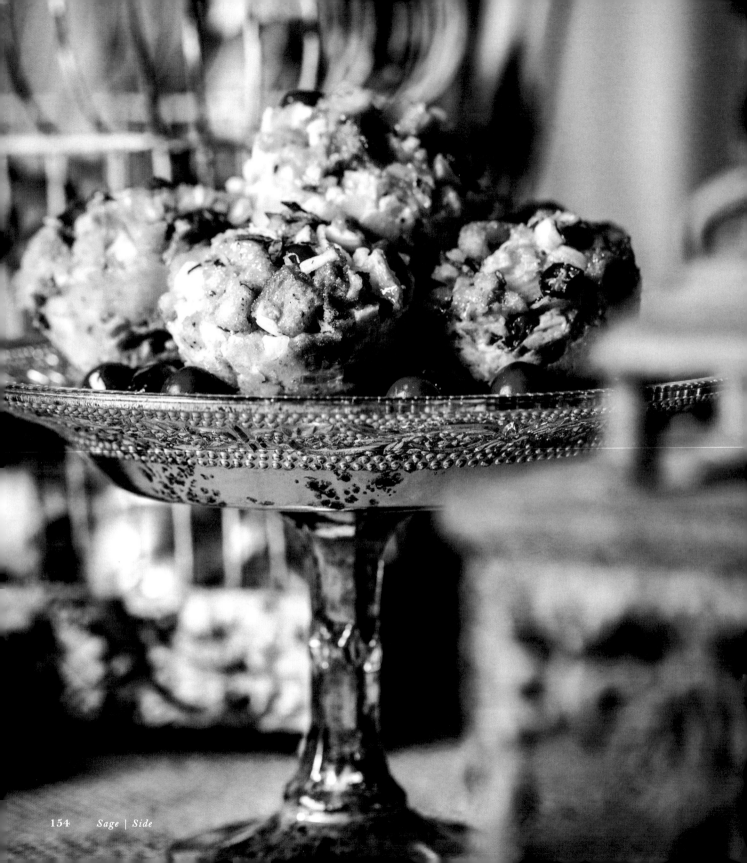

CRANBERRY SAGE STUFFINS

Although sage in stuffing is as common as peanut butter with jelly, a sage chapter without some kind of stuffing recipe just seems wrong. These individual stuffing muffins are easy to make and very flavorful. The added crunch due to their smaller size is an added bonus. To make life easier on Thanksgiving, stuffins can be made in muffin cups, stored in containers overnight, and reheated just before serving.

2 large eggs, beaten

¼ cup reduced-sodium chicken broth

¼ cup fresh apple cider

1 Tbsp. unsalted butter, melted

⅓ cup chopped apple

⅓ cup diced onion

¼ cup chopped celery

¼ cup fresh cranberries, halved

2 Tbsp. finely chopped fresh sage leaves, loosely packed

1 Tbsp. chopped fresh parsley leaves

½ tsp. poultry seasoning

1 cup dry stuffing mix

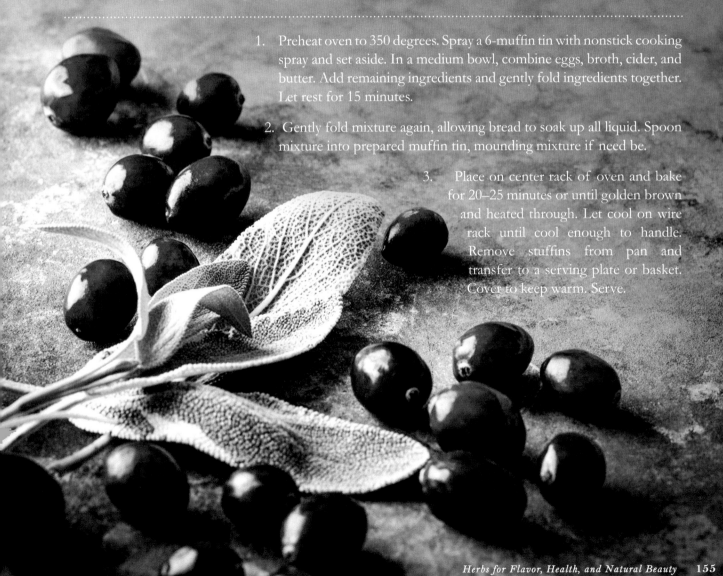

1. Preheat oven to 350 degrees. Spray a 6-muffin tin with nonstick cooking spray and set aside. In a medium bowl, combine eggs, broth, cider, and butter. Add remaining ingredients and gently fold ingredients together. Let rest for 15 minutes.

2. Gently fold mixture again, allowing bread to soak up all liquid. Spoon mixture into prepared muffin tin, mounding mixture if need be.

3. Place on center rack of oven and bake for 20–25 minutes or until golden brown and heated through. Let cool on wire rack until cool enough to handle. Remove stuffins from pan and transfer to a serving plate or basket. Cover to keep warm. Serve.

PORCHETTA RIBS WITH BALSAMIC GLAZE

The flavor of the fresh sage and rosemary really sings in this modern day twist to a classic tuscan dish. You may never want traditional barbecued ribs again. It works equally well with baby back ribs or boneless pork roast.

2 tsp. fennel seeds

½ tsp. red pepper flakes

½ tsp. black pepper, freshly ground

3 Tbsp. EVOO

½ cup water

2 Tbsp. white balsamic vinegar

¼ cup fresh sage leaves, chopped

2 Tbsp. fresh rosemary leaves, chopped

1 Tbsp. fresh parsley, chopped

3 cloves garlic, minced

1 tsp. kosher salt

1 rack pork spareribs, cut into individual ribs

16 slices pancetta

1. Toast fennel seeds and next three ingredients In a small skillet over medium heat for 1–2 minutes or until lightly browned, shaking pan to keep spices from burning. Remove from heat and let cool completely. Transfer mixture to a spice grinder or clean coffee grinder. Grind to a fine powder. Transfer mixture to a 1-gallon re-sealable plastic bag.

2. Add remaining ingredients except ribs and pancetta to the bag of spices. Seal and shake bag to combine ingredients. Open bag and add ribs one at a time. Seal bag, removing as much air as possible. Move ribs around in bag until they are well coated with marinade. Place bag in a 13- X 9- in. baking dish. Refrigerate for 4–8 hours or overnight.

3. Preheat oven to 325 degrees. Drain marinade from ribs. Transfer ribs to the same baking dish. Cover with aluminum foil. Bake for 1 hour or until meat is tender. Remove ribs from oven and let them cool to room temperature.

4. Increase oven temperature to 425 degrees. Wrap one slice of pancetta around each cooked rib. Roast ribs uncovered for 15–20 minutes or until ribs are browned and pancetta is crispy. Brush ribs with balsamic glaze and return to oven. Bake an additional 5–10 minutes. Remove from oven and serve.

SERVINGS: 4 | SOURCE: Little Rusted Ladle

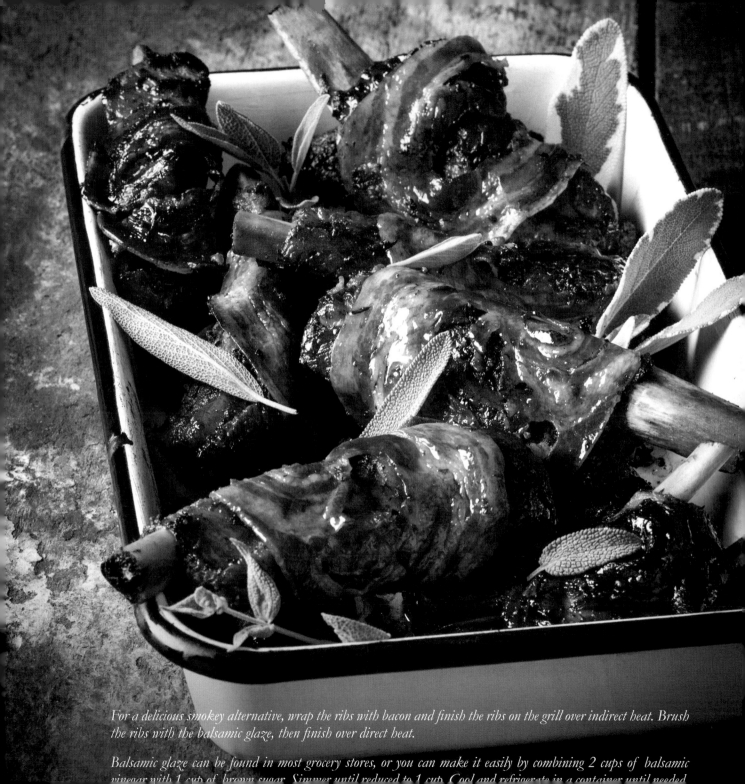

For a delicious smokey alternative, wrap the ribs with bacon and finish the ribs on the grill over indirect heat. Brush the ribs with the balsamic glaze, then finish over direct heat.

Balsamic glaze can be found in most grocery stores, or you can make it easily by combining 2 cups of balsamic vinegar with 1 cup of brown sugar. Simmer until reduced to 1 cup. Cool and refrigerate in a container until needed.

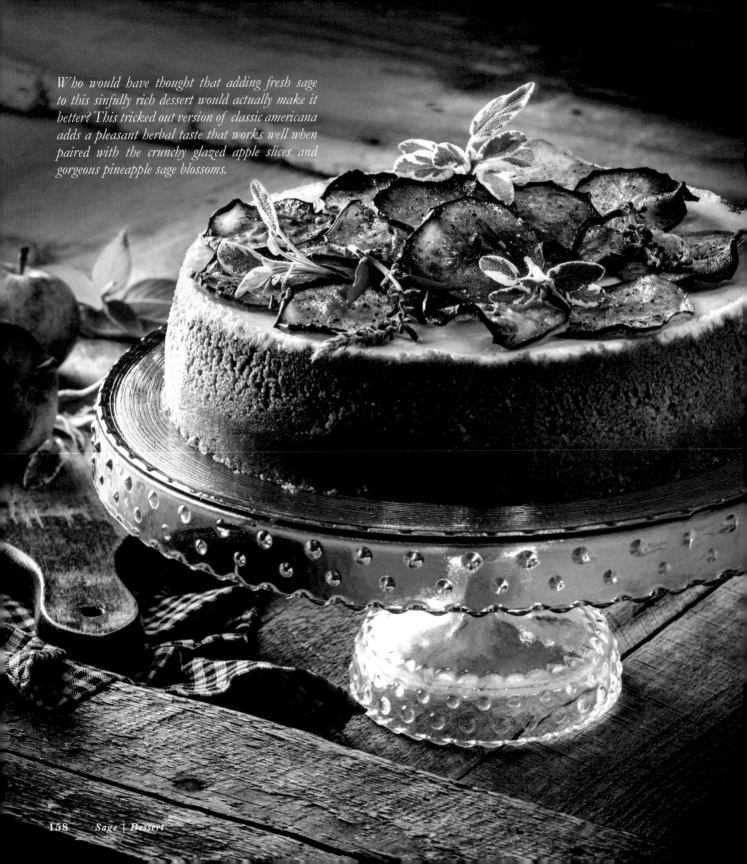

Who would have thought that adding fresh sage to this sinfully rich dessert would actually make it better? This tricked out version of classic americana adds a pleasant herbal taste that works well when paired with the crunchy glazed apple slices and gorgeous pineapple sage blossoms.

MAPLE & SAGE CHEESECAKE WITH APPLES & SAGE BLOSSOMS

1½ cups graham cracker crumbs

½ cup chopped walnuts

3 Tbsp. sugar

¼ tsp. kosher salt

4 Tbsp. unsalted butter, melted

24 oz. cream cheese, softened

¾ cup sugar

4 large eggs

2 Tbsp. flour

1 cup sour cream

½ cup pure maple syrup, divided

2 Tbsp. fresh lemon juice

Hot water

¼ cup fresh sage leaves, cut crosswise into thin strips

¼ cup fresh pineapple sage leaves, cut crosswise into thin strips

2 fresh apples, thinly sliced

¼ tsp. cinnamon

1. FOR CRUST, preheat oven to 375 degrees. Combine graham cracker crumbs and next three ingredients in a food processor. Pulse 4–5 times or until nuts are finely ground. Add butter and pulse another 4–5 times. Spray the inside of a 9-inch springform pan with nonstick spray. Transfer crumb mixture to pan. Press crumbs into the bottom and up sides using a flat drinking glass. Bake for ten minutes or until light golden brown. Remove and let cool while making filling. Reduce oven temperature to 325 degrees.

2. FOR FILLING, in a large mixing bowl, beat cream cheese and sugar on medium-low speed until smooth. Add eggs one at a time, scraping down bowl after each egg. Add flour, sour cream, half of maple syrup, and lemon juice. Beat until smooth. Pour over cooled crust. Place a large piece of heavy-duty foil in a large roasting pan. Place filled springform pan on top of foil. Add hot water to roasting pan until it is halfway up springform pan. Bring up sides of foil to prevent water from getting cheesecake wet. Place in oven. Add hot water to roasting pan until it is halfway up springform pan. Bake for 80–90 minutes or until center of cheesecake is almost set. Remove from oven and transfer cheesecake to a rack. Let cool to room temperature. Cover and refrigerate overnight.

3. FOR APPLES, place apple slices on a sheet pan lined with nonstick foil. Brush apple slices with remaining maple syrup and sprinkle with cinnamon. Bake at 450 degrees for 10–12 minutes. Turn apple slices over with a fork. Brush slices with maple syrup. Place a small sage leaf on top of slices, then brush remaining syrup over sage leaves. Broil on top rack for 3–4 minutes or until syrup has caramelized and apples are browned. Transfer apples to a wire rack to cool.

4. TO ASSEMBLE, carefully remove cheesecake from pan by releasing lever. Run knife around edge if it sticks. Transfer cheesecake to a plate. Stack apple slices on top of cheesecake. Garnish with fresh sage leaves and pineapple sage flowers if desired.

SERVINGS: 8 | SOURCE: Little Rusted Ladle

STRAWBERRY SAGE SHRUB

Shrubs have been around for centuries and are making a triumphant comeback thanks to the craft cocktail craze at restaurants. The vinegar adds nice acidity that gives it that refreshing quality, and the fresh sage gives it the herbal notes that make it complete. Serve it over ice or use it as a mixer with your favorite libation.

2 cups water

1 cup sugar

2 cups apple cider vinegar

4 cups fresh strawberries, hulled and sliced

2 sprigs fresh sage, washed

1. Combine water and sugar in a medium saucepan over medium heat. Simmer for 3–4 minutes or until sugar dissolves.

2. Stir in strawberries and cook an additional ten minutes. Add vinegar and cook an additional two minutes.

3. Remove from heat and stir in sage. Let cool for one hour at room temperature.

4. Strain mixture into a glass container with a lid. Store in refrigerator for up to two weeks or until needed.

SERVINGS: 4
SOURCE: Little Rusted Ladle

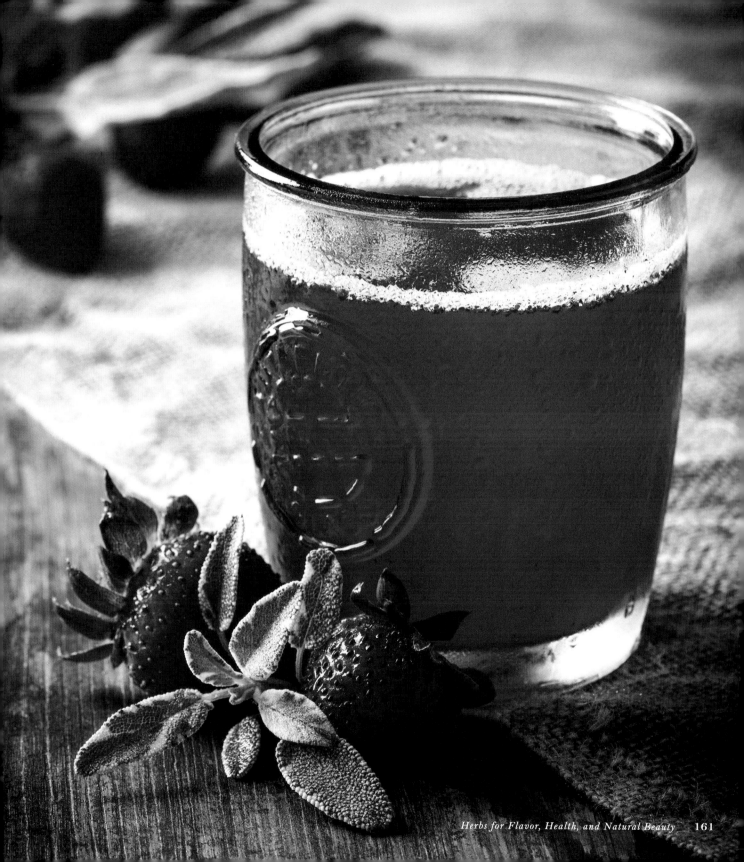

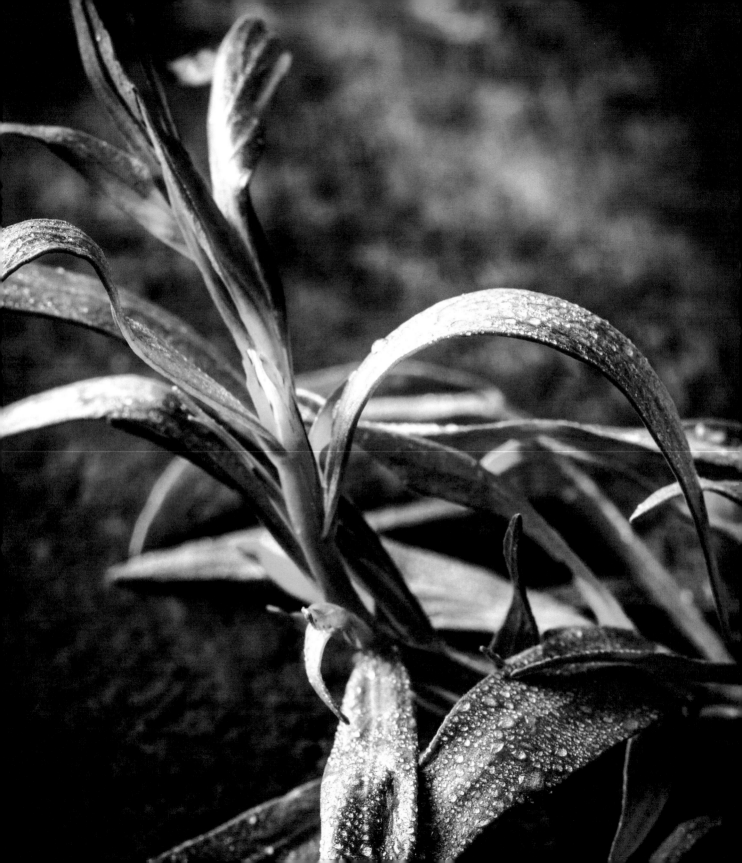

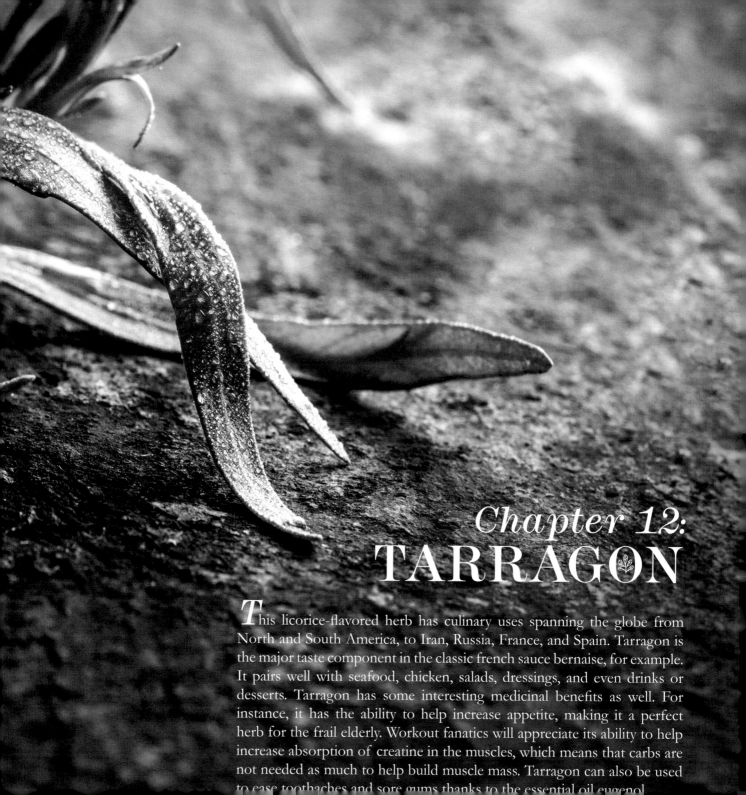

Chapter 12:
TARRAGON

*T*his licorice-flavored herb has culinary uses spanning the globe from North and South America, to Iran, Russia, France, and Spain. Tarragon is the major taste component in the classic french sauce bernaise, for example. It pairs well with seafood, chicken, salads, dressings, and even drinks or desserts. Tarragon has some interesting medicinal benefits as well. For instance, it has the ability to help increase appetite, making it a perfect herb for the frail elderly. Workout fanatics will appreciate its ability to help increase absorption of creatine in the muscles, which means that carbs are not needed as much to help build muscle mass. Tarragon can also be used to ease toothaches and sore gums thanks to the essential oil eugenol.

GRILLED LOBSTER TAILS WITH TARRAGON CHIVE BUTTER

The flavor of fresh tarragon combined with the chive blossom butter from page 43 is the perfect compliment to fresh lobster tails. This very simple recipe takes less than 15 minutes to make, but the taste will last a lifetime. Feel free to serve this dish as a main course over pasta or simply brush the butter over swordfish, grouper, or any other firm, fresh fish.

1. Preheat gas or charcoal grill. Split lobster tails down the middle lengthwise with a sharp knife. Remove middle vein. Place lobster halves on a sheet pan or baking dish flesh-side up.

2. Melt butter in a small saucepan until just melted. Add tarragon and stir to combine. Brush melted tarragon butter liberally over lobster meat. Place lobster tails on grill over direct heat. Grill for 7–10 minutes or until lobster meat is white in color.

3. Carefully remove from grill, being careful not to let melted butter in tails to drip out of shell. Brush with additional butter if desired and serve as an appetizer with lemon wedges.

3 lobster tails, 6–8 oz. each

2 Tbsp. chive blossom butter or unsalted butter, see Chive Blossom Butter recipe on page 43

2 Tbsp. chopped fresh tarragon

Salt and pepper to taste

Lemon wedges, optional

SERVINGS: 4 | SOURCE: Little Rusted Ladle

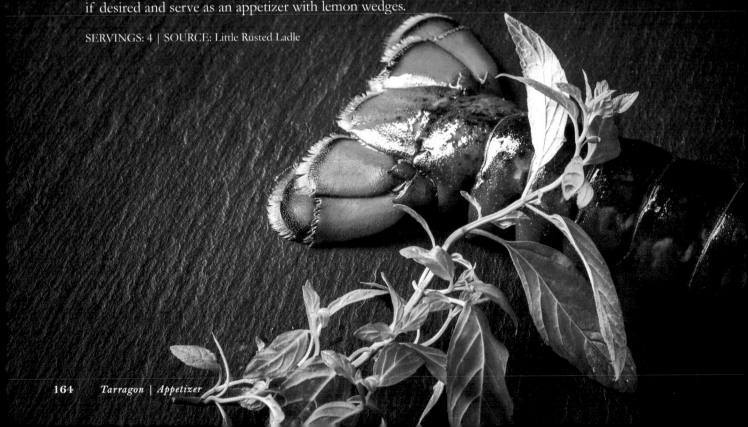

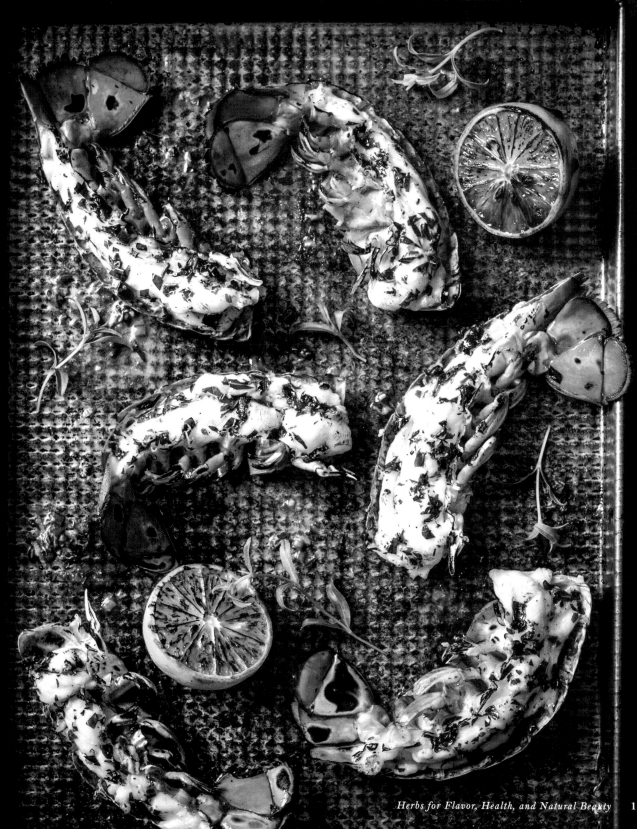

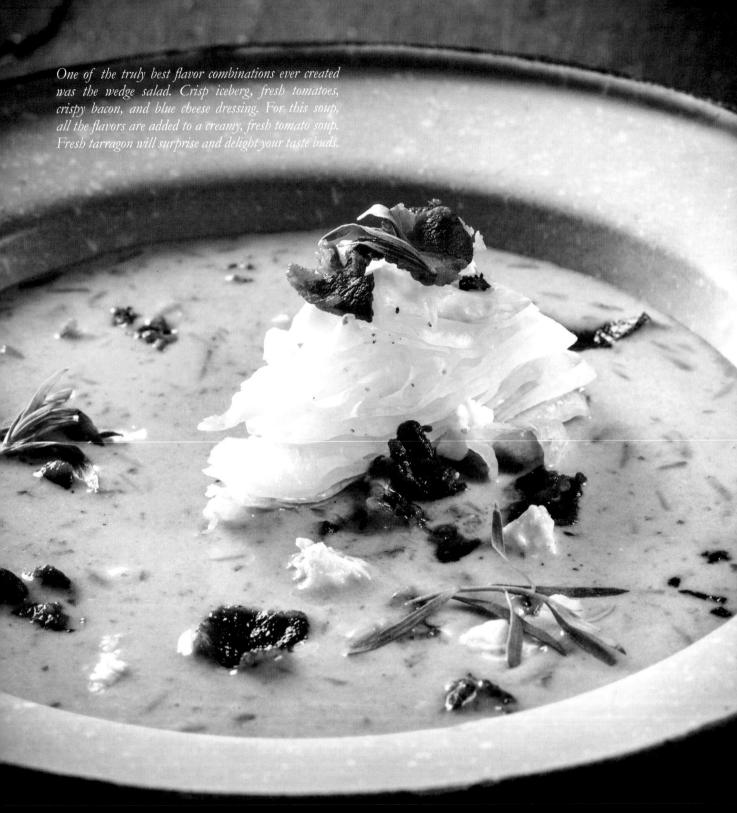

One of the truly best flavor combinations ever created was the wedge salad. Crisp iceberg, fresh tomatoes, crispy bacon, and blue cheese dressing. For this soup, all the flavors are added to a creamy, fresh tomato soup. Fresh tarragon will surprise and delight your taste buds.

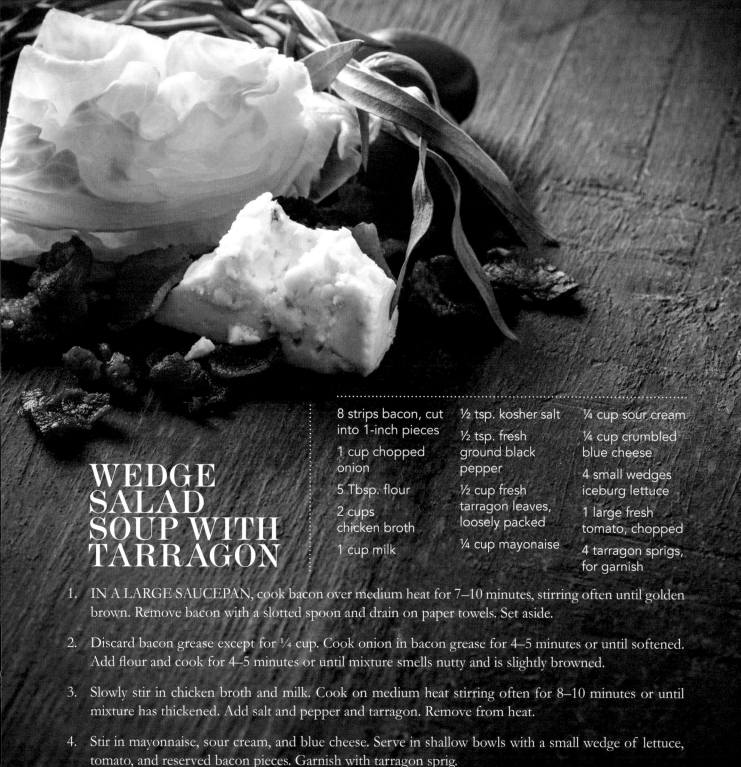

WEDGE SALAD SOUP WITH TARRAGON

8 strips bacon, cut into 1-inch pieces

1 cup chopped onion

5 Tbsp. flour

2 cups chicken broth

1 cup milk

½ tsp. kosher salt

½ tsp. fresh ground black pepper

½ cup fresh tarragon leaves, loosely packed

¼ cup mayonaise

¼ cup sour cream

¼ cup crumbled blue cheese

4 small wedges iceburg lettuce

1 large fresh tomato, chopped

4 tarragon sprigs, for garnish

1. IN A LARGE SAUCEPAN, cook bacon over medium heat for 7–10 minutes, stirring often until golden brown. Remove bacon with a slotted spoon and drain on paper towels. Set aside.

2. Discard bacon grease except for ¼ cup. Cook onion in bacon grease for 4–5 minutes or until softened. Add flour and cook for 4–5 minutes or until mixture smells nutty and is slightly browned.

3. Slowly stir in chicken broth and milk. Cook on medium heat stirring often for 8–10 minutes or until mixture has thickened. Add salt and pepper and tarragon. Remove from heat.

4. Stir in mayonnaise, sour cream, and blue cheese. Serve in shallow bowls with a small wedge of lettuce, tomato, and reserved bacon pieces. Garnish with tarragon sprig.

SERVINGS: 4 | SOURCE: Little Rusted Ladle

SPICY TARRAGON PICKLES

These pickles are a tribute to those classic jumbo pickles fermented in barrels at local grocery stores. For this version though, I decided to use vinegar instead of letting them naturally ferment at room temperature as the ones in the barrels usually are. Tarragon replaces the expected dill. Since I love spicy pickles, 4 different levels of hot peppers were added along with garlic, salt, sugar, and, of course, pickling spice. Feel free to use smaller cucumbers, eliminate the hot peppers, or try them with different herbs like chive blossoms, basil, or a combination of herbs. There are no rules, just suggestions. Enjoy.

2 qt. water

3 cups water

2 cups white vinegar

1 cup apple cider vinegar

1 cup sugar

⅓ cup pickling salt

2 Tbsp. pickling spice

4 garlic cloves, crushed

4 fresh tarragon sprigs

6 jumbo pickling cucumbers, ends cut off

4 fresh red and green jalapeños pepper, sliced ½-inch thick

2 fresh habanero peppers, sliced

1 hot banana pepper, sliced ½-inch thick

1 serrano pepper, sliced

1. TO STERILIZE JAR, bring 2 quarts of water to a boil in a large saucepan or stockpot. Pour boiling water into a large, clean glass jar or container (2 quart). Leave water in container for ten minutes, then pour water out of container. Set aside.

2. TO MAKE BRINE, in a large saucepan, combine 3 cups water and next six ingredients. Bring to a boil, reduce heat and simmer for five minutes or until sugar is dissolved. Remove from heat. Transfer brine to a 4-cup heat-proof glass pitcher.

3. TO MAKE PICKLES, place 2 sprigs of tarragon in the bottom of the jar. Pack cucumbers and peppers in the jar. Add remaining tarragon. Pour hot brine over pickles to an inch below the top. Cover and let cool completely. Store in refrigerator for at least ten days before eating. Eat within four weeks.

SERVINGS: 12 | SOURCE: Little Rusted Ladle

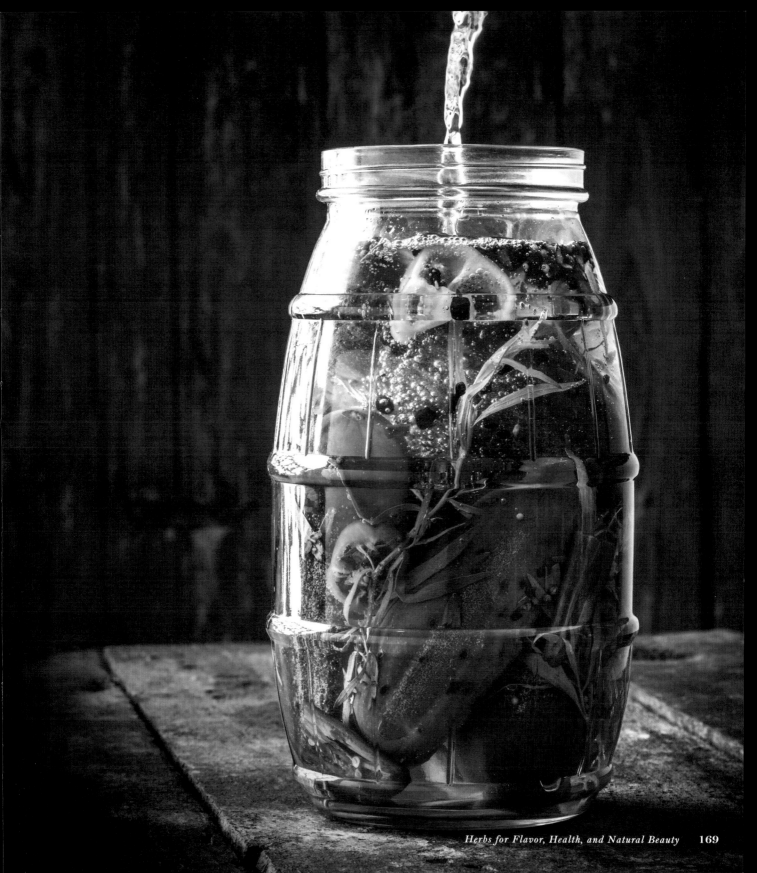

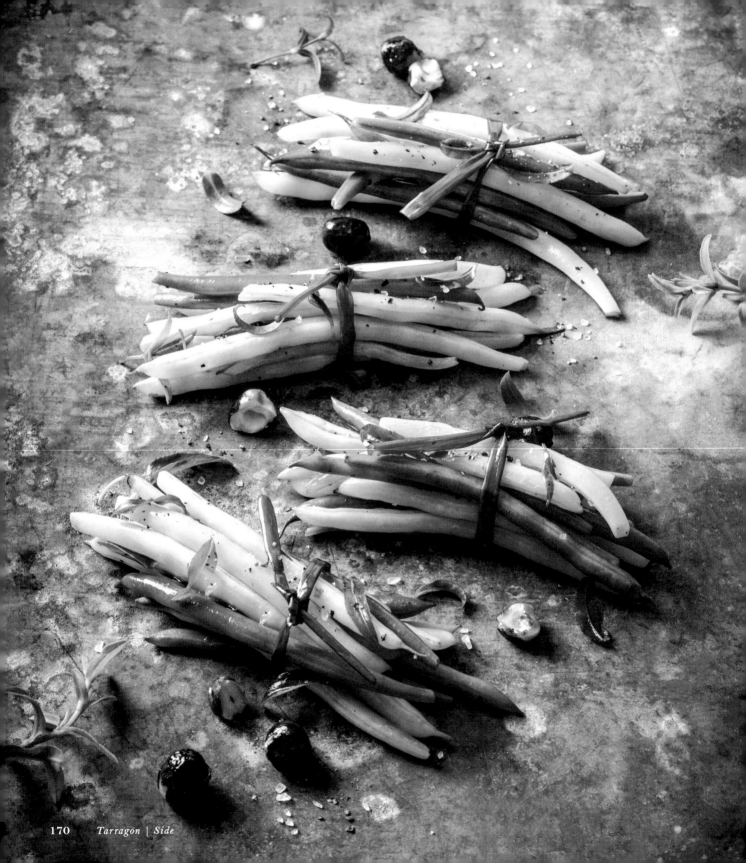

BEAN BUNDLES WITH FRESH TARRAGON & GLAZED HAZELNUTS

Fresh pole beans out of the garden remind me of my childhood. To this day, I still love the squeak of the beans while eating them. This recipe gives the standard pole bean a facelift by adding the wonderful anise flavor of fresh tarragon and sweet glazed hazelnuts. Fresh chives are used to create cute little bundles of yum. Your family will think they are in a gourmet restaurant. Feel free to omit the chives and serve them in a bowl when you just want beans to be simple.

⅓ cup hazelnuts

1 Tbsp. light brown sugar

1 Tbsp. apple cider

2 tsp. coconut oil

¼ lb. fresh waxed beans, trimmed

¼ lb. fresh green beans, trimmed

2 Tbsp. chopped fresh mexican tarragon leaves

Salt and pepper to taste

4 chives

Tarragon leaves, for garnish

1. FOR HAZELNUTS, in a small skillet over medium heat, toast hazelnuts for 3–4 minutes, shaking pan often. Add brown sugar and apple cider. Shake pan to melt sugar and coat nuts. Continue to move the pan back and fourth while the mixture cooks and reduces to a syrupy glaze, about two minutes. When nuts are well-coated and mixture is the consistency of caramel, dump nuts onto a small sheet pan lined with foil. Let nuts cool completely, then break nuts up and set aside.

2. FOR BEANS, in a large nonstick skillet over medium heat, melt coconut oil. Add beans and sauté for 5–7 minutes or until crisp-tender. Mix in tarragon leaves. Season with salt and pepper. Place one chive on a cutting board. Using a pair of tongs, transfer 7–8 cooked beans over the center of the chive. Bring ends of chive up over beans and tie into a knot. Repeat with remaining chives and beans. Serve with glazed hazelnuts and tarragon leaves for a garnish.

SERVINGS: 4 | SOURCE: Little Rusted Ladle

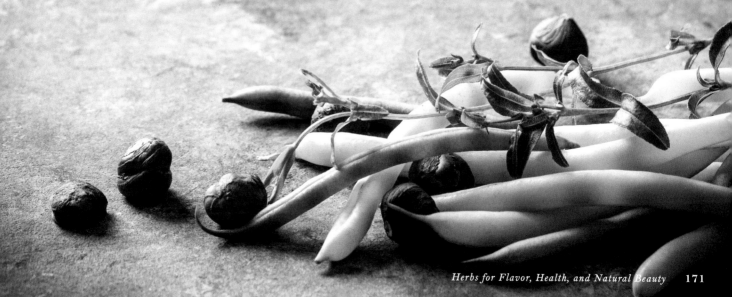

APPLE & FENNEL BRINED PORK CHOPS

2 qt. cold water

½ cup fine sea salt

1 cup fresh apple cider

½ cup real maple syrup

1 Tbsp. dried fennel seed

½ cup diced onion

1 tsp. crushed red pepper flakes

4 cloves garlic, chopped

2 sprigs fresh parsley

5 ea. fresh tarragon sprigs

2 sprigs fresh thyme

2 sprigs fresh sage

4 8–12-oz. bone-in pork rib chops

2 tsp. curry powder

1 tsp. dried basil

½ tsp. crushed red pepper flakes

3 strips applewood smoked bacon, cut into ½ inch pieces

1 small red onion, cut into strips

3 small parsnips, peeled and halved lengthwise

¼ cup fresh cranberries

2 cloves garlic, chopped

8 large brussels sprouts, separated into leaves

1. **TO BRINE PORK CHOPS**, combine water and next 11 ingredients in a 4-quart container with a lid. Stir, then let sit until salt dissolves. Stir again, then add pork chops, making sure liquid covers meat. Cover and refrigerate for 4–8 hours or overnight.

2. **TO SEASON PORK CHOPS**, remove pork chops from brine and pat dry with paper towels. In a small bowl, combine curry powder, basil, and red pepper flakes. Rub mixture over pork chops. Let rest at room temperature for 15 minutes while cooking bacon.

3. **TO COOK PORK CHOPS**, preheat oven to 375 degrees. Transfer brined pork chops to a plate and dry with paper towels. In a large, heavy bottomed skillet or frying pan, cook bacon over medium heat until browned. Transfer bacon to a small plate, leaving remaining bacon grease in pan to brown pork chops. When bacon is removed from pan, add pork chops and parsnips to pan with bacon grease. Cook over medium heat for 4–5 minutes per side or until golden brown. Transfer chops to a plate and set aside. Add apple cider to pan with parsnips and scrape up any brown bits with a spatula.

4. Transfer parsnips and pan drippings to a small roasting pan or shallow baking dish. Add onions and cranberries to pan with parsnips. Add any juices from pork and toss to coat. Roast in oven for 30 minutes. Remove from oven, place pork chops over vegetables, add brussels sprouts leaves and return to oven. Roast an additional 10–15 minutes or until vegetables are tender and pork is slightly firm to the touch and cooked to medium. Remove from oven. Serve topped with cooked bacon.

SERVINGS: 4

SOURCE: Little Rusted Ladle

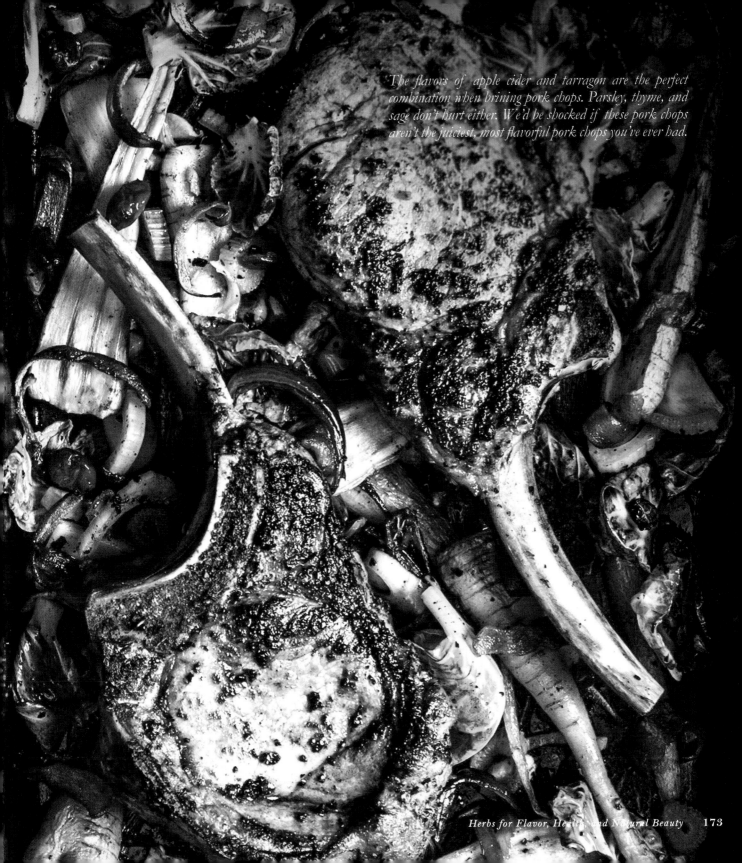

The flavors of apple cider and tarragon are the perfect combination when brining pork chops. Parsley, thyme, and sage don't hurt either. We'd be shocked if these pork chops aren't the juiciest, most flavorful pork chops you've ever had.

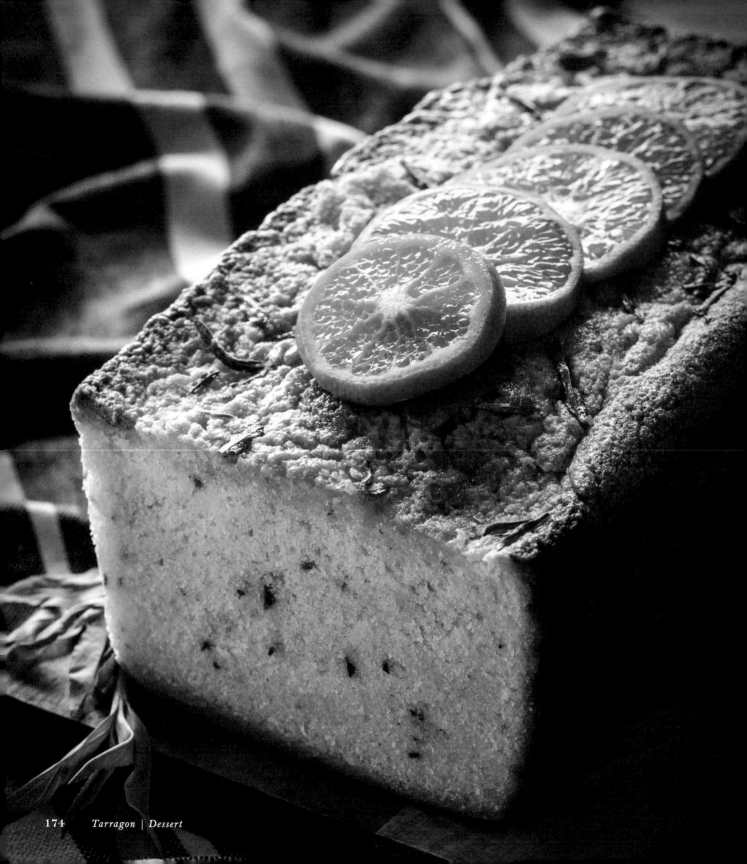

TARRAGON POUND CAKE WITH CLEMENTINE GLAZE

Buttery pound cake, flavored with fresh tarragon, then bathed in a sweet clementine vanilla glaze. What a perfect way to showcase this licorice-flavored herb. Feel free to add chocolate chips, nuts, or dried fruit to the batter before baking.

....

2 sticks unsalted butter, room temperature	Mexican tarragon leaves	1 oz. fresh clementine juice from 1 clementine
1½ cups sugar	1 tsp. baking powder	4 Tbsp. sugar
3 oz. cream cheese, room temperature	2 tsp. vanilla extract	2 tsp. chopped fresh mexican tarragon leaves
2 Tbsp. finely chopped fresh	5 large eggs	1 tsp. vanilla extract
	1¾ cups unbleached flour	

1. Preheat oven to 350 degrees. In a large mixing bowl, combine butter and next five ingredients. Beat on medium speed for one minute or until light and fluffy.

2. With motor running, add eggs one at a time and beat on medium speed for 30 seconds each time. When all eggs have been added, beat an additional three minutes.

3. Add flour slowly until mixture is creamy. Pour into a greased 9 x 5 x 2 ¾ loaf pan. Place on center rack. Bake for 30 minutes.

4. FOR CLEMENTINE GLAZE, while cake is baking, in a small bowl, combine clementine juice and remaining ingredients. Set aside until cake has baked for 30 minutes.

5. Remove cake from oven. Brush top with clementine glaze, making sure to add the leaves as well. Return pan to oven and bake an additional 15 minutes or until golden brown. Remove pan from oven. Let cool for ten minutes, then carefully remove cake from pan and place on a cooling rack. Poke holes in top of cake with a toothpick or cake tester. Brush top with remaining clementine glaze. Let cool completely. Serve.

SERVINGS: 6 | SOURCE: Little Rusted Ladle

TARRAGON ICED TEA WITH PINEAPPLE

Ice tea on a hot summer day can really quench your thirst. This version simply adds fresh pineapple and tarragon to give it a little extra pizzazz. If you like your tea a little sweeter, stir in ¼ cup honey at the same time as the pineapple and tea bags. For you Arnold Palmer fans, fill a glass half full with the tea, then top it with the Thyme Pink Lemonade Recipe on page 192.

5 cups water

5 tea bags of your choice

2 cups cut into chunks fresh pineapple

6 large fresh tarragon sprigs

1. IN A LARGE SAUCEPAN, bring water to a low simmer. Remove from heat and add tea bags and pineapple. Let cool completely, then add mixture to a pitcher or carafe. Add tarragon. Refrigerate for at least four hours or overnight. Serve over ice.

SERVINGS: 4 | SOURCE: Little Rusted Ladle

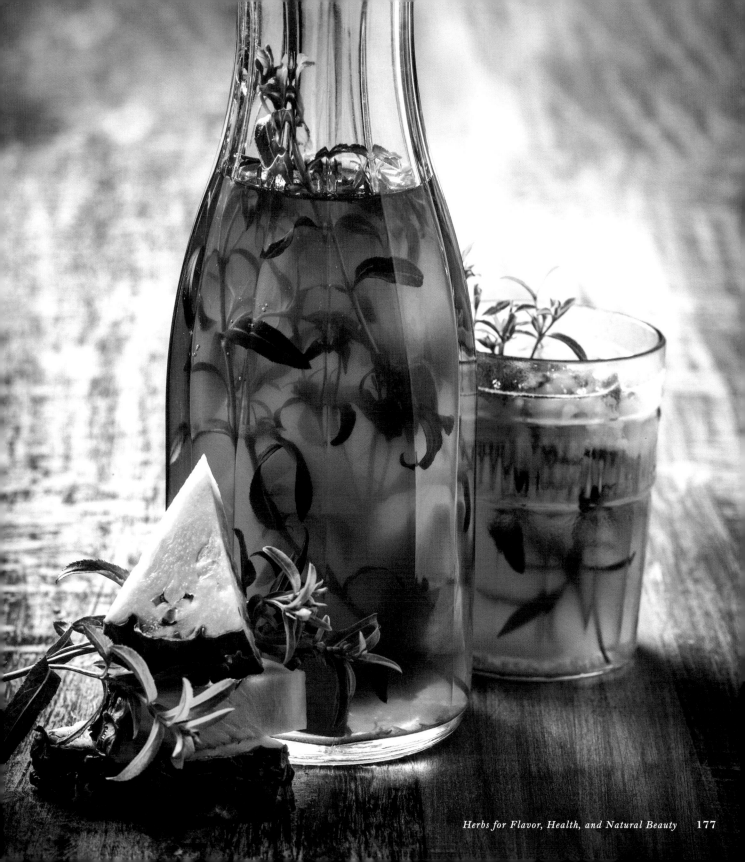

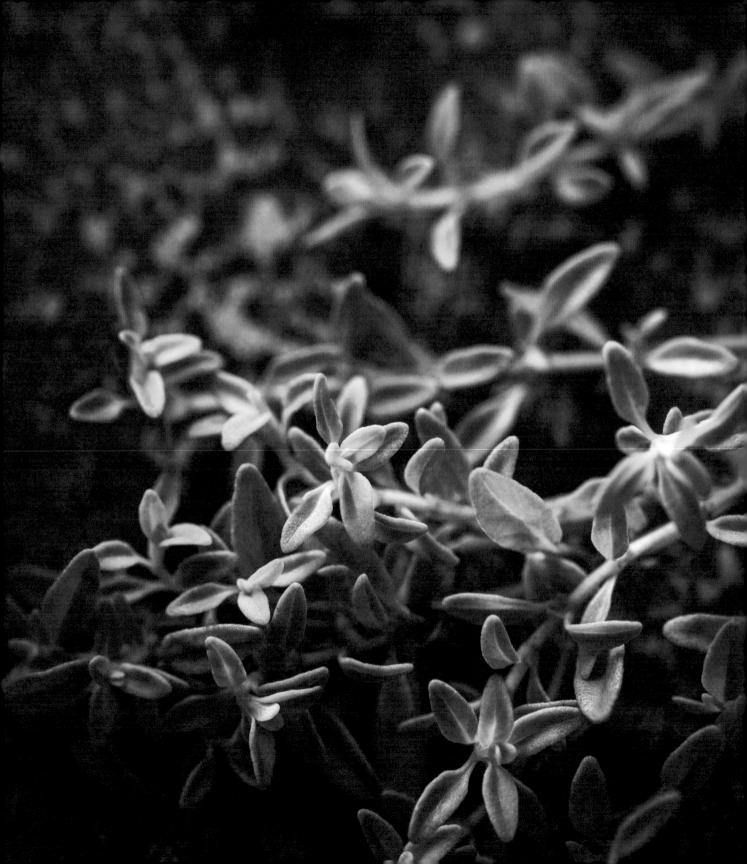

Chapter 13:
THYME

*T*hyme is one of those herbs that find its way into so many countries, cultures, and culinary classic recipes that it's hard to think of cooking without it. Can you imagine standard seasonings like bouquet garni, jerk seasoning, herbs de provence, cajun, or zaatar seasoning without thyme? Yet each of these seasonings is used in completely different cultures with extremely different flavors. Pretty indispensable, if you ask me. Another wonderful quality of thyme is how diverse its flavor can be. In dried form, it is wonderfully intense, giving soups, meats, and dressings their distinct flavor. In fresh form, it is completely different, which can vary on the variety. French and english thyme are the most common and most flavorful to use in the kitchen, but lemon thyme is another great option. Thyme isn't just known for its culinary prowess. Its medicinal properties have been used since the ancient Egyptians used thyme in the mummification process. Other uses include being used to eliminate bad odors, helping eliminate parasites in the body, treating the common cold or whooping cough, cleaning the skin, and even repelling insects while bringing in bees which pollinate plants. Wow, that's a beneficial herb!

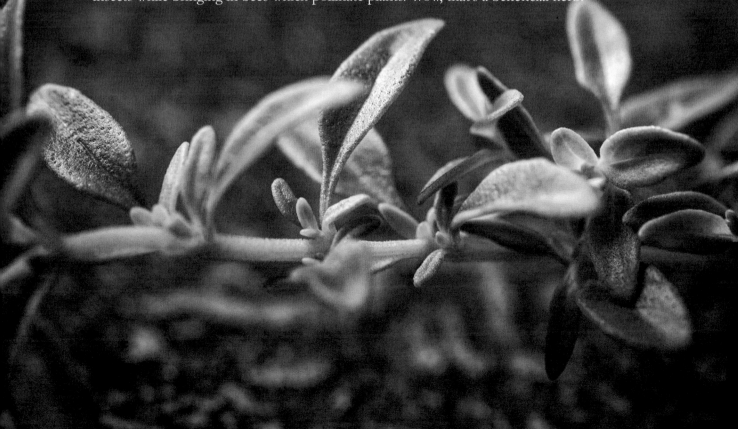

BACON-WRAPPED FIGS WITH GORGONZOLA & THYME HONEY

Fresh figs in the summer are one of my favorite fruits. They are so beautiful and when they are ripe, they are so sweet. However, when you add some musty gorgonzola and wrap it in bacon with fresh thyme, they take on a completely different kind of yummy. Exclude the bacon and they are almost as good. Almost.

¼ cup raw honey

1 Tbsp. fresh thyme leaves

4 fresh figs, cut in half lengthwise

3 Tbsp. gorgonzola cheese

8 sprigs fresh thyme

4 slices smoked bacon, cut in half

Fresh ground black pepper

1. Preheat oven to 375 degrees. Place bacon on a rack over a foil-lined sheet pan. Bake for 10 minutes or until most of the bacon grease has been rendered. Drain on paper towels and let cool.

2. FOR THYME HONEY, prepare honey by warming honey in a small saucepan. Add thyme leaves. Keep warm over low heat for 4–5 minutes. Transfer honey to a small bowl and set aside to cool.

3. TO ASSEMBLE FIGS, spoon a half a tablespoon into the cut side of each fig half. Place 1 sprig of thyme over cheese. Wrap one bacon half around fig and fasten with a toothpick. Repeat with remaining figs. Place wrapped figs on the same sheet pan. Sprinkle pepper over bacon. Roast figs for 7–8 minutes. Brush with reserved thyme honey. Roast an additional 7–8 minutes or until bacon is golden brown. Drizzle with more thyme honey and serve.

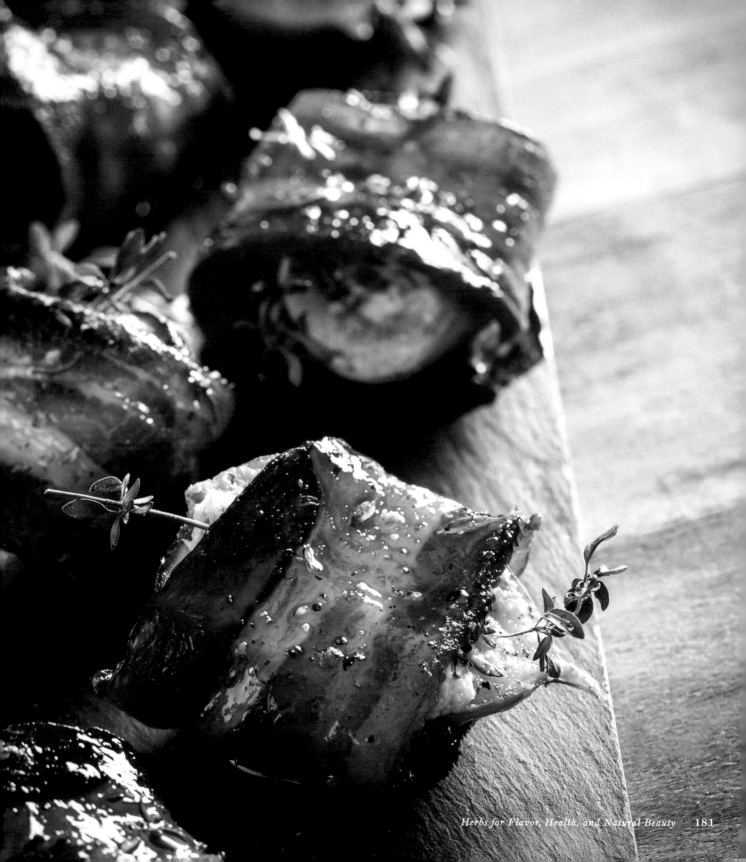

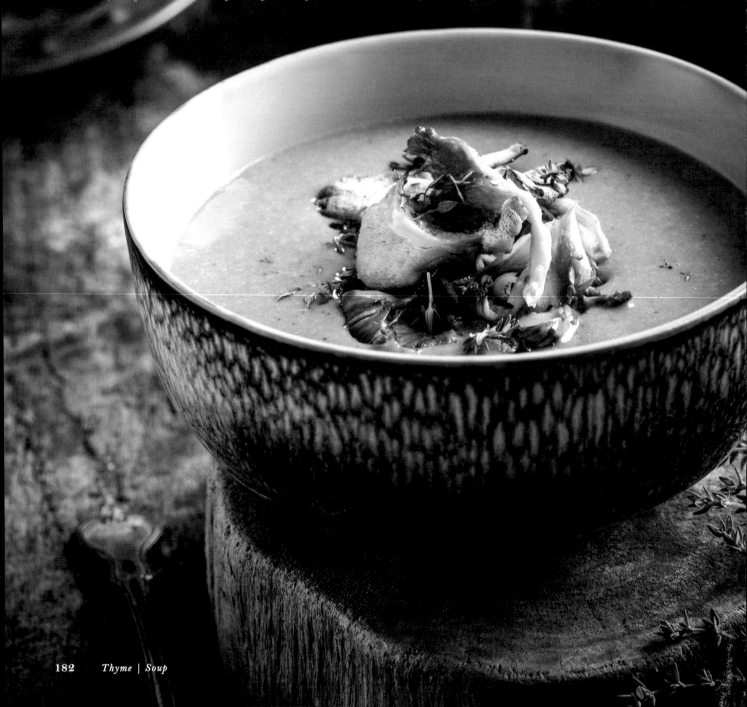

Every season different wild mushrooms start popping in the forest. Unlike the ones found in the grocery stores, these mushrooms have much different flavors. From morels in the spring to chanterelles in the summer to maitake mushrooms in the fall. The one thing they all have in common is they taste great in soup and are delicious with fresh thyme. If you cannot find wild mushrooms near you, the soup is designed to be great without needing to add them on top. Wild mushrooms like morels, chanterelles, and maitake (hen of the woods) can often be found at farmers markets throughout the spring, summer, and fall months.

WILD MUSHROOM & THYME BISQUE

3 Tbsp. unsalted butter

½ cup sweet onion, diced

1 cup button mushrooms, sliced

1 cup crimini mushrooms, sliced

2 cloves garlic, minced

¼ cup fresh thyme leaves, divided

4 Tbsp. flour

2 cups chicken stock

1 cup half-and-half, warmed

1 cup canned pumpkin

Salt and pepper to taste

2 cups wild mushrooms (morel, maitake, oyster, chanterelle, etc.), cut into large chunks

1 Tbsp. EVOO

1 tsp. Kosher salt

1. TO MAKE SOUP, melt butter over medium heat in a larges saucepan. Add onions and mushrooms. Sauté for 3–4 minutes or until softened, stirring once or twice. Add garlic and half of thyme leaves. Cook an additional 3–4 minutes until liquid has reduced by half. Stir in flour. Cook for 3–4 minutes or until mixture has thickened. Stir in chicken stock, half-and-half, and pumpkin. Reduce heat to simmer and cover and cook for 20 minutes, stirring occasionally until soup is hot and has thickened. Season to taste with salt and pepper. Keep warm while roasting mushrooms.

2. TO PREPARE WILD MUSHROOMS, preheat oven to 425 degrees. Line a baking sheet with foil. Place mushrooms on pan and drizzle with oil. Season with salt and pepper. Roast mushrooms for 12–15 minutes or until cooked through and edges are crispy. Remove from oven and set aside until ready to serve.

3. TO SERVE, stir in remaining thyme leaves just before serving. Ladle into bowls and top with roasted mushrooms. Sprinkle with additional thyme leaves if desired. Serve immediately. Enjoy.

SERVINGS: 4 | SOURCE: Little Rusted Ladle

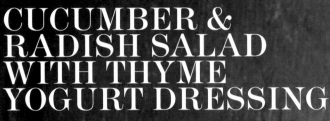

CUCUMBER & RADISH SALAD WITH THYME YOGURT DRESSING

Fresh cucumber salad with sour cream dressing was always a favorite of my parents while growing up. This version adds radishes, an assortment of fresh herbs, and substitutes greek yogurt for the sour cream. The nasturtiums add an additional peppery flavor similar to watercress.

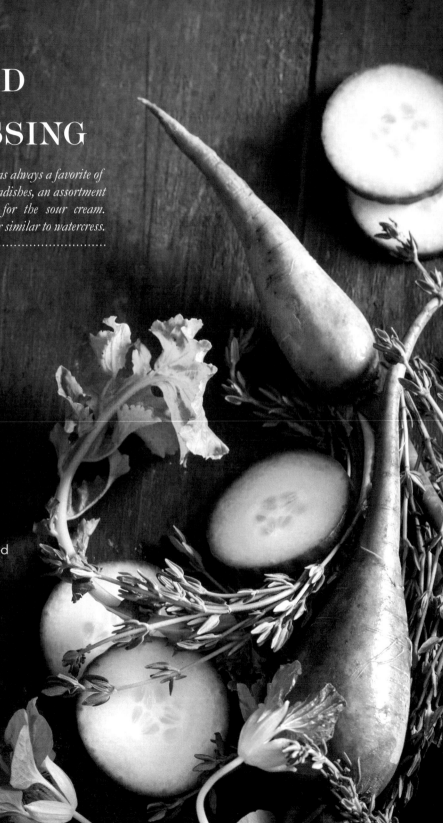

½ cup greek yogurt

½ tsp. fresh horseradish

½ tsp. garlic, minced

1 Tbsp. honey

2 tsp. fresh lemon juice

½ tsp. kosher salt

1 Tbsp. chopped fresh chives

2 tsp. chopped fresh parsley

1 Tbsp. chopped fresh thyme leaves

2 cups thinly sliced fresh purple radishes

2 cups thinly sliced seedless cucumbers

Fresh ground black pepper

2 Tbsp. fresh nasturtium leaves

2 fresh nasturtium flowers, petals removed

Fresh thyme leaves for garnish, optional

1. IN A LARGE BOWL, combine yogurt and next eight ingredients. Add radishes and cucumbers. Toss to coat. Sprinkle with nasturtium leaves and petals, pepper, and thyme. Serve.

SERVINGS: 4 | SOURCE: Little Rusted Ladle

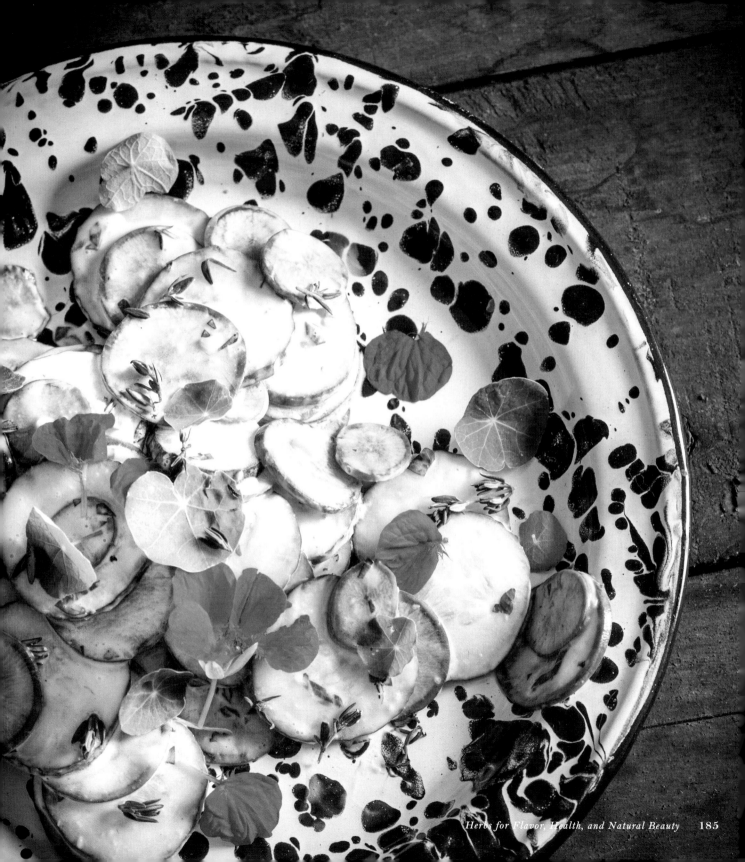

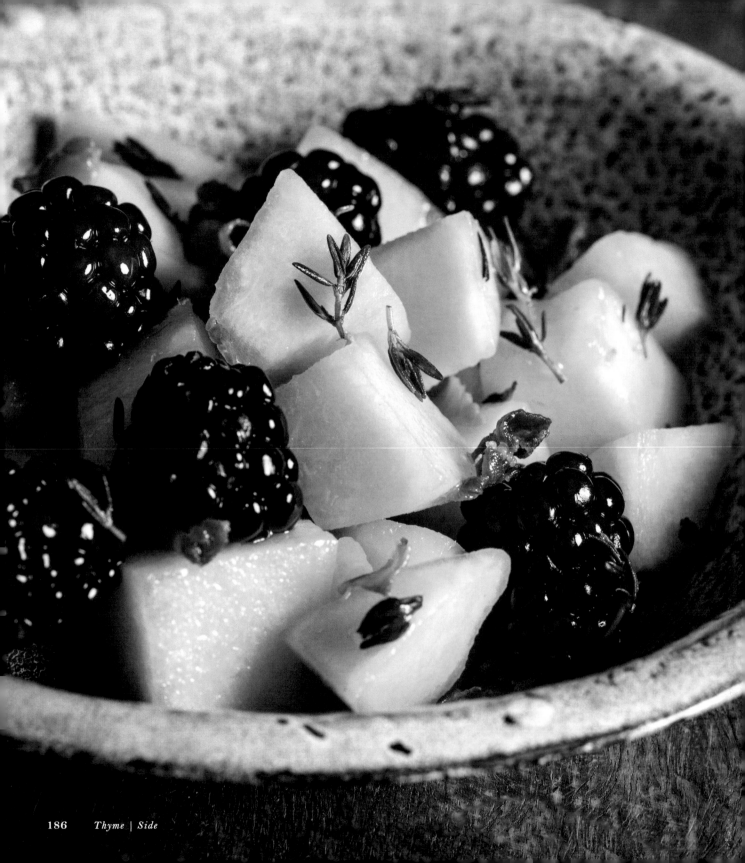

MELON & BLACKBERRY SALAD WITH FRIED PROSCUITTO & THYME

It's no wonder melon and prosciutto are a classic combination. For this Italian tribute, fresh blackberries are added with a lemon thyme oil used to fry the prosciutto, which adds crunch and that irresistible salty element that makes this salad so delicious.

1. FOR PROSCIUTTO, in a small skillet, heat oil over low heat until warm. Add lemon peels and half of thyme. Cook over low heat for ten minutes. Remove peels and thyme. Turn heat up to medium. When temperature is 300–350 degrees, carefully add prosciutto. Fry until golden brown. Remove from heat and transfer prosciutto to a plate with a slotted spoon. Let remaining lemon oil in pan (about 1 tablespoon) cool to room temperature. Set aside.

2. FOR SALAD, in a medium size bowl, gently combine melon, blackberries, remaining thyme, fried prosciutto, and reserved lemon oil (1 tablespoon).

SERVINGS: 4 | SOURCE: Little Rusted Ladle

2 Tbsp. light olive oil

1 oz. prosciutto, diced

2 pieces lemon peel

1½ Tbsp. chopped fresh thyme leaves, divided

2 cups cubed fresh cantaloupe melon

2 cups fresh blackberries

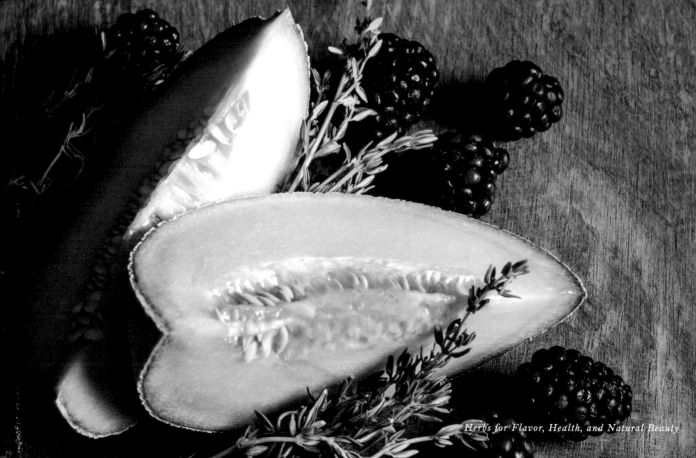

DOUBLE THYME JERK CHICKEN PIZZA

Jerk chicken pizza may not sound like a very nice name for a recipe, but don't let the name fool you. This pizza is very complex, thanks in large part to the intense flavors of fresh thyme, allspice, habanero peppers, and soy sauce. These ingredients infuse the chicken with a sweet, savory heat that will wake up your taste buds. If you'd rather just eat the chicken, go right ahead. Nobody will blame you for not waiting.

1 cup chopped onion

¾ cup soy sauce

½ cup distilled white vinegar

¼ cup vegetable oil

¼ cup light brown sugar

2 Tbsp. chopped fresh thyme leaves

1 habanero pepper, cut in half

6–8 chives, chopped

1 tsp. ground allspice

½ tsp. fresh ground nutmeg

¼ tsp. ground cloves

4 boneless, skinless chicken thighs

2 par-baked pizza crusts

3 cups mozzarella cheese, shredded

2 cups quesadilla cheese, shredded

1 cup small, sweet pepper rings

1 cup cut into strips red onion

½ cup diced fresh mango

1 Tbsp. chopped fresh thyme leaves

FOR JERK MARINADE, in a blender, combine onion and next ten ingredients. Blend on high until almost smooth. Transfer half of marinade to a resealable plastic bag. Add chicken thighs, remove as much air as possible, then seal and refrigerate at least four hours or overnight. Refrigerate remaining marinade in a container until ready to assemble pizza.

FOR CHICKEN, preheat grill to medium heat. Remove chicken from marinade, removing as much marinade as possible. Grill chicken for 5–7 minutes on each side over direct heat until cooked through and juices run clear. Let chicken cool completely. Meanwhile, prepare pizza.

TO MAKE PIZZA, preheat oven to 400 degrees. Spread reserved jerk marinade on pizza crusts. Divide cheese, cooled chicken, and remaining ingredients on sauced crusts. Bake for 12–15 minutes or until cheese has melted and crust is golden brown. Cut into wedges and serve.

SERVINGS: 4 | SOURCE: Little Rusted Ladle

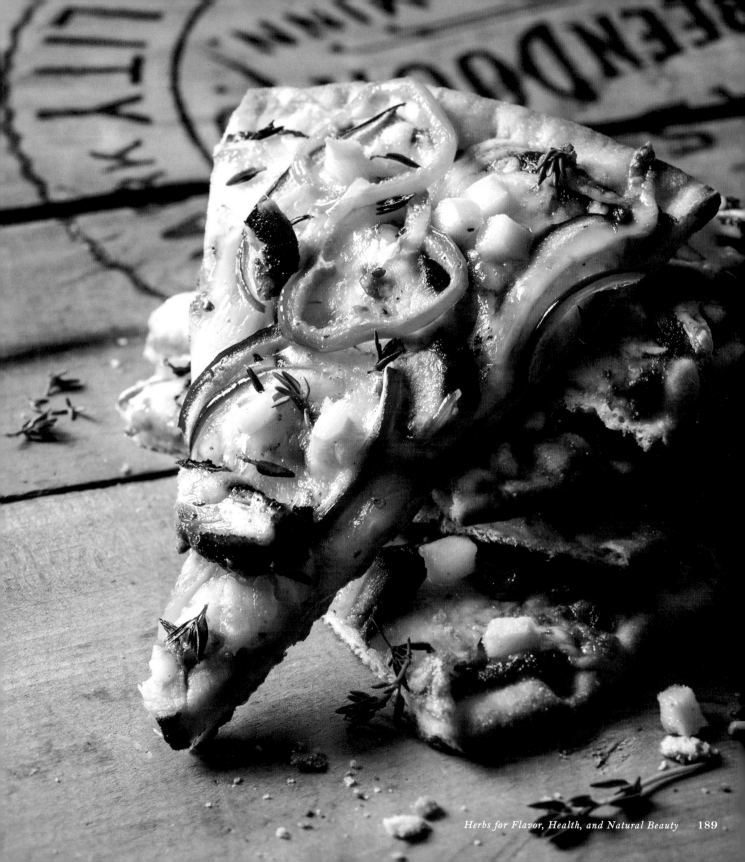

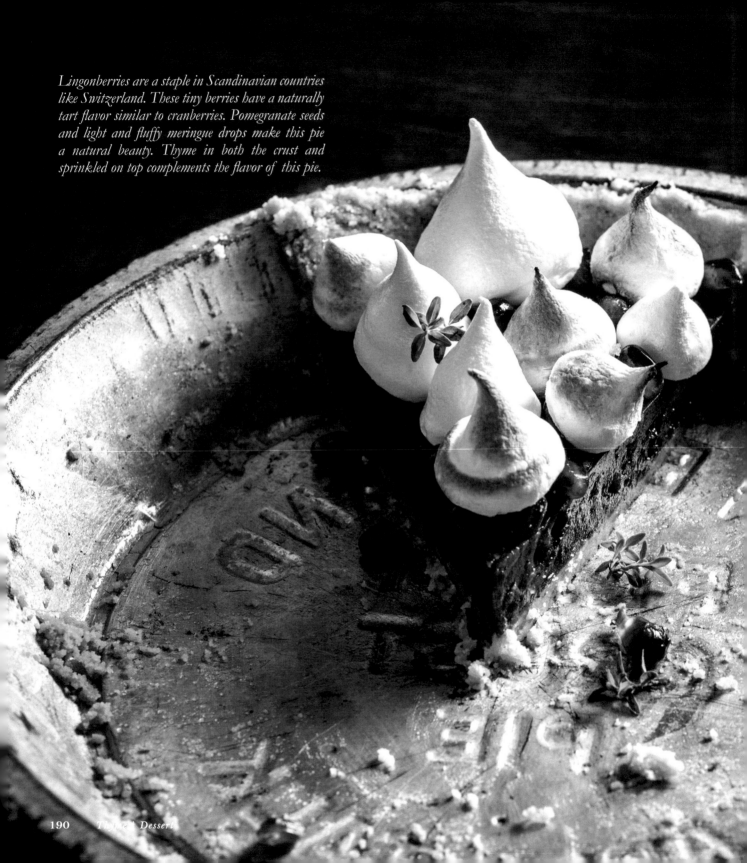

Lingonberries are a staple in Scandinavian countries like Switzerland. These tiny berries have a naturally tart flavor similar to cranberries. Pomegranate seeds and light and fluffy meringue drops make this pie a natural beauty. Thyme in both the crust and sprinkled on top complements the flavor of this pie.

LINGONBERRY MERINGUE PIE WITH THYME SHORTBREAD CRUST

1 (5.3 oz.) package
shortbread cookies

1 Tbsp. chopped fresh
thyme leaves

2 Tbsp. sugar

2 Tbsp. unsalted
butter, melted

2 envelopes
unflavored gelatin

¼ cup pomegranate
juice

2 cups lingonberry
preserves

¼ cup sour cream

3 large egg whites,
room temperature

1 tsp. pure vanilla extract

¼ tsp. cream of tartar

1 pinch salt

⅔ cup sugar

½ cup pomegranate
arils (seeds), divided

1 tsp. chopped fresh
lemon or lime thyme
leaves for garnish

1. FOR THYME SHORTBREAD CRUST, combine shortbread cookies and next three ingredients in the bowl of a food processor. Pulse 8–10 times or until cookies are finely ground. Transfer mixture to a shallow 8-inch pie plate. Press crumbs into bottom and up sides using a flat-bottomed drinking glass. Bake for ten minutes or until golden brown. Cool crust completely. Refrigerate until ready to fill.

2. FOR LINGONBERRY FILLING, in a small bowl, combine gelatin and cranberry juice. Let gelatin bloom for 5 minutes. Meanwhile, in a medium saucepan, melt lingonberries reserves over medium low heat. Stir in gelatin. Cook on low until gelatin has melted into lingonberries. Remove from heat and transfer mixture to a glass or metal bowl. Place bowl over a larger bowl of ice water. Slowly stir mixture until lingonberries start to thicken. Pour into prepared crust. Refrigerate until gelatin has firmed up.

3. FOR TOASTED MERINGUE DROPS, preheat oven to 250 degrees. Combine egg whites and next three ingredients in a large mixing bowl. Beat on medium speed until foamy. Slowly add sugar, beating once or twice until sugar is dissolved. Beat on medium for 6–8 minutes or until glossy, stiff peaks form.

4. Transfer meringue to a resealable plastic bag with a 1-inch hole cut out of the bottom corner. Line a sheet pan with parchment paper. Pipe meringue into ¾ x 1¼ drops 2 inches apart. Broil half of drops in oven until lightly browned on top. Bake for 45 minutes. Turn off oven and leave meringues in oven for one hour or until firm to the touch. Cool completely.

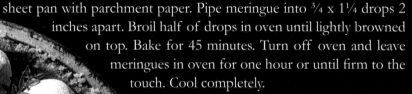

5. TO ASSEMBLE PIE, remove pie from refrigerator. Sprinkle pomegranate arils over lingonberry mixture. Top with cooled meringue drops, more pomegranate arils, and fresh thyme leaves. Serve.

SERVINGS: 6 | SOURCE: Little Rusted Ladle

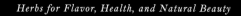

THYME PINK LEMONADE

This version of the popular summer classic is a lot better for you than that powdery mix from the store. It's super easy to make and you don't have to waste all that time juicing lemons. The thyme and cranberry add a wonderful bouquet of flavor and add that beautiful red color that comes from nature, not a laboratory. By blending the whole lemon into the drink, you get added fiber, vitamins, and all the health benefits that go with it. You will get more juice and less pith if you use lemons that are very ripe when you buy them. A ripe lemon is soft when squeezed. When you cut the lemon, you will see a much thinner skin. Buy organic lemons when possible, and be sure to scrub the lemons well before using.

1 cup cranberries, fresh or frozen

5 cups water, divided

1½ cups sugar or honey

3 bunches fresh thyme, divided

4 organic lemons, washed and quartered

4 lemon slices, for garnish

1. Combine cranberries, 1½ cup water, sugar, and 2 bunches of thyme in a medium saucepan. Simmer 3–5 minutes, stirring occasionally, until sugar dissolves and cranberries pop. Strain mixture into a pitcher through a fine sieve. Refrigerate until cool.

2. Meanwhile, combine remaining water and lemon quarters in a blender. Blend on high until cloudy and lemons are in little pieces. Strain into cooled cranberry syrup and stir until well blended. Refrigerate until cold. Serve over ice with a sprig of thyme and a lemon slice for garnish.

SERVINGS: 4 | SOURCE: Little Rusted Ladle

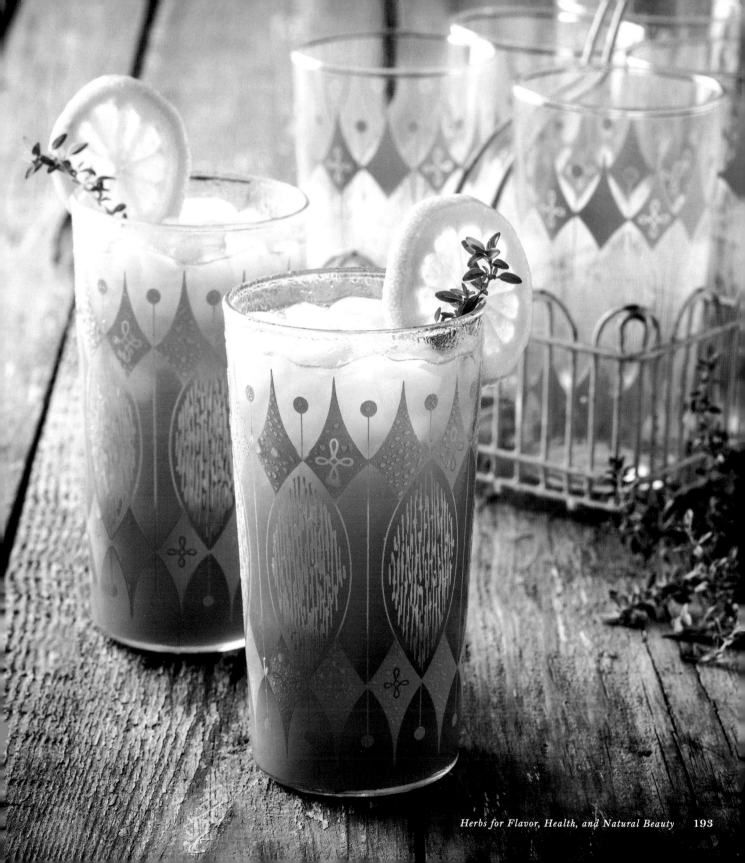

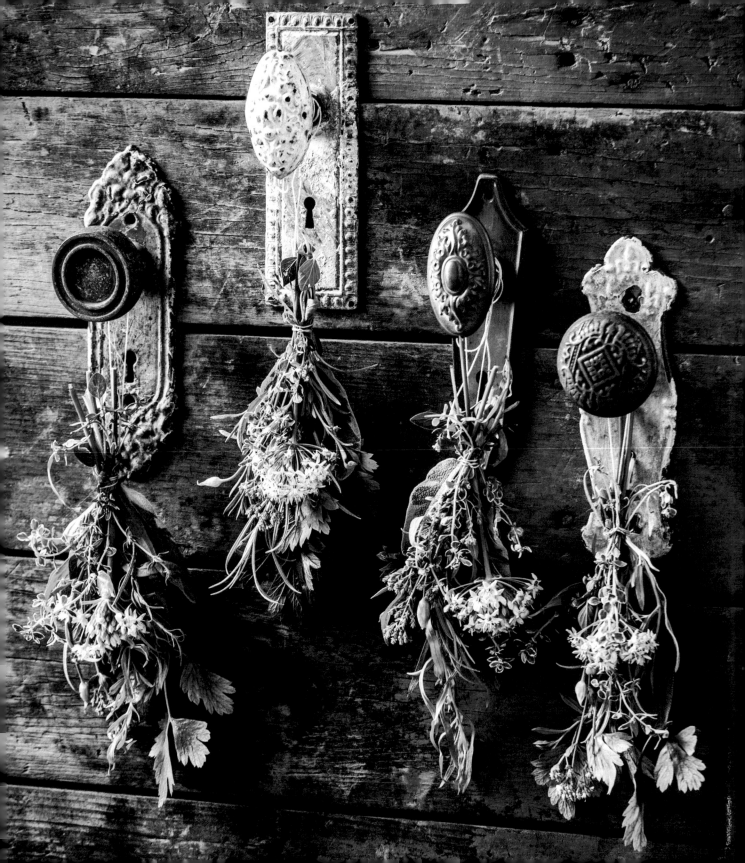

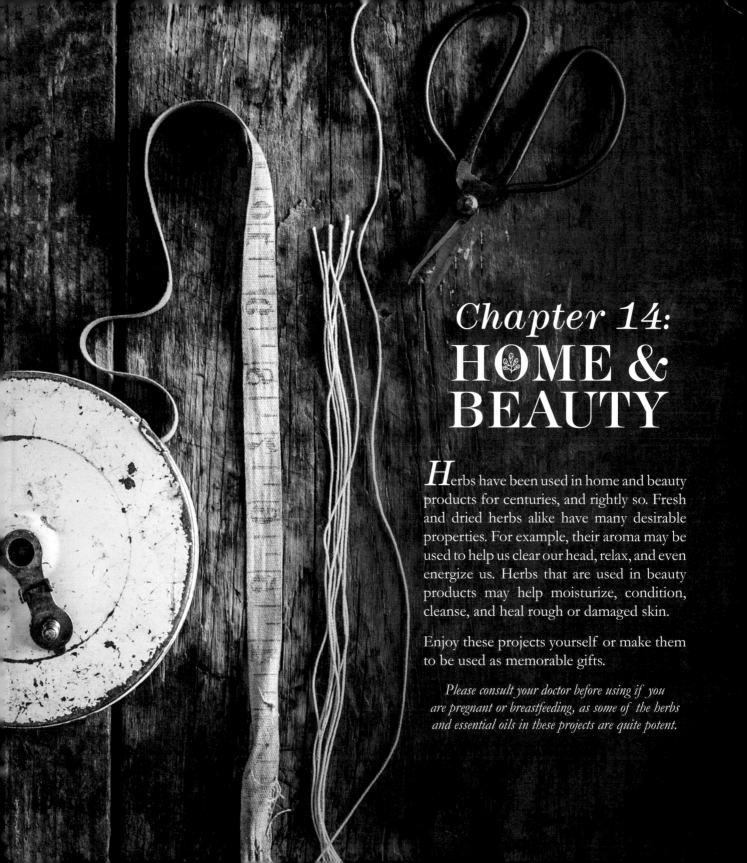

Chapter 14:
HOME & BEAUTY

*H*erbs have been used in home and beauty products for centuries, and rightly so. Fresh and dried herbs alike have many desirable properties. For example, their aroma may be used to help us clear our head, relax, and even energize us. Herbs that are used in beauty products may help moisturize, condition, cleanse, and heal rough or damaged skin.

Enjoy these projects yourself or make them to be used as memorable gifts.

Please consult your doctor before using if you are pregnant or breastfeeding, as some of the herbs and essential oils in these projects are quite potent.

FRESH HERB WREATH

Fill your home with this timeless trio of lavender, rose, and eucalyptus. This fresh lavender, rose, and eucalyptus wreath is just as beautiful dried, with its gently faded colors and lingering scent.

6 mini bouquets lavender

Floral wire

6 sprigs of eucalyptus

6 light purple roses

Metal wreath form

1. Make lavender bouquets with about ten sprigs of lavender and hold together with floral wire.

2. Take one eucalyptus sprig, place one lavender bouquet in front of it, then place one rose in front of the lavender bouquet, making sure that you are able to view each of the three items. Wrap the items together with wire and then attach them to the wire wreath holder.

3. Repeat these steps all the way around the wreath.

Note: The fresh wreath only lasts a day or two, so to extend its beauty and usefulness you should dry the items.

Instructions for drying: Use crumpled newsprint to support the heavy heads of the roses and to preserve the shape of the wreath. Lay the wreath face up somewhere it can be left undisturbed until completely dry – generally about 2-3 days. Rehang the wreath when dry. Add a few drops of essential oil.

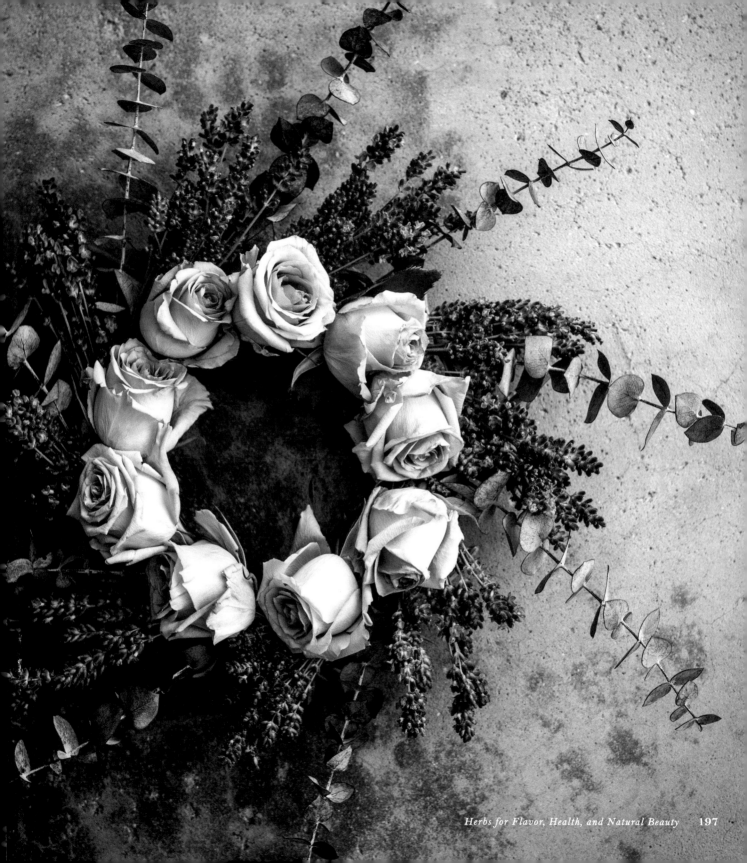

For our dried soup gift, we made a mini herbal wreath
to tie on the front of the jar. The mini wreath is meant
to be used in the soup itself. This recipe makes one jar.

DRIED HEARTY ITALIAN BEAN SOUP GIFT

FOR THE HERB WREATH

6 basil leaves

6 parsley leaves

6 sprigs of oregano

6 sprigs of rosemary

6 sprigs of thyme

Floral Wire

Wire circle—about the size of a quarter.

2½ cup size glass jar or larger

THE HEARTY ITALIAN BEAN SOUP

¼ cup white beans

¼ cup garbanzo beans

¼ cup kidney beans

2 Tbsp. chicken stock bouillon

¼ cup dried onion

¼ cup sundried tomatoes

½ tsp. black pepper

½ tsp. garlic powder

1. Make six tiny bouquets of basil, parsley, oregano, rosemary, and thyme using one piece of each herb. Wire them together at the base.

2. Wrap each bouquet on the wire circle with wire, overlapping one another and filling the circle.

3. Tie a bouquet onto the jar containing the rest of the soup mix.

1. Layer all of the ingredients in the jar.

2. Add the wreath and instructions to the tag.

INSTRUCTIONS TO PUT ON THE TAG

1. Bring four cups of water to a simmer.

2. Remove the herbs from the metal ring.

3. Add the contents of jar and herbs.

4. Stir to resolve bouillon.

5. Cook until the beans are softened—normally around four hours.

HERBAL TEA SWAGS

Host the perfect tea party with your homemade tea swags! These swags are tied with cotton kitchen string and are able to hold themselves together, so there is no need for a traditional tea bag. Just infuse hot water with these aromatic bundles and serve. It's an herb garden in a teapot!

8 leaves lemon verbena

8 sprigs lavender

8 leaves mint

8 sprigs rosemary

8 sprigs basil

Lengths of 100% cotton kitchen twine

1. Bundle and tie 1–2 pieces of each sprig and leaf together.

2. Tie tags to the tea swags.

3. Hang the tea swags upside down to dry for about two weeks, or they can be used fresh.

4. Add to hot water, steep for 3–5 minutes.

MAKES 4 CUPS

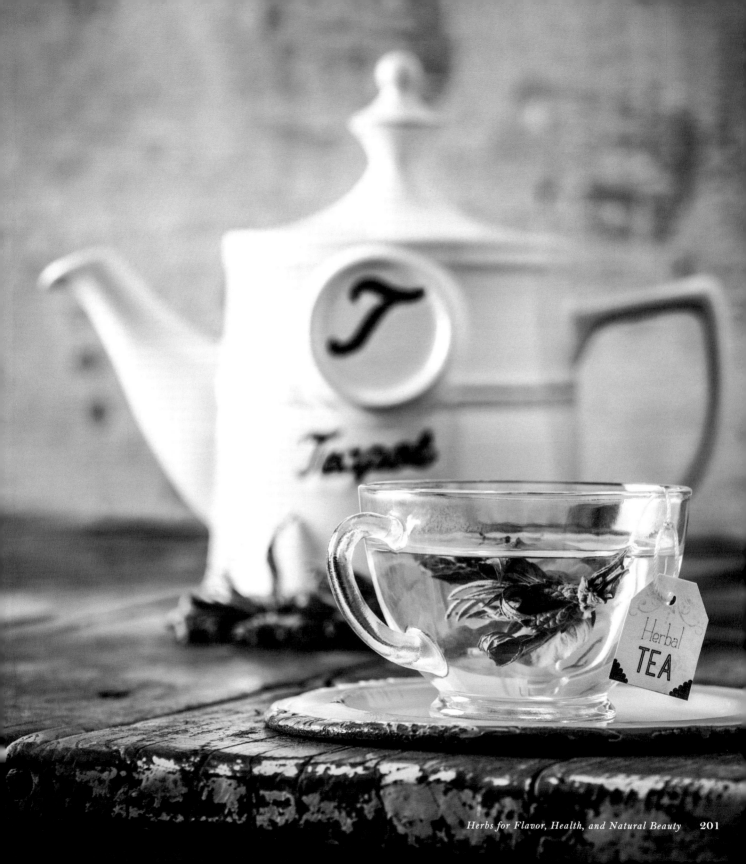

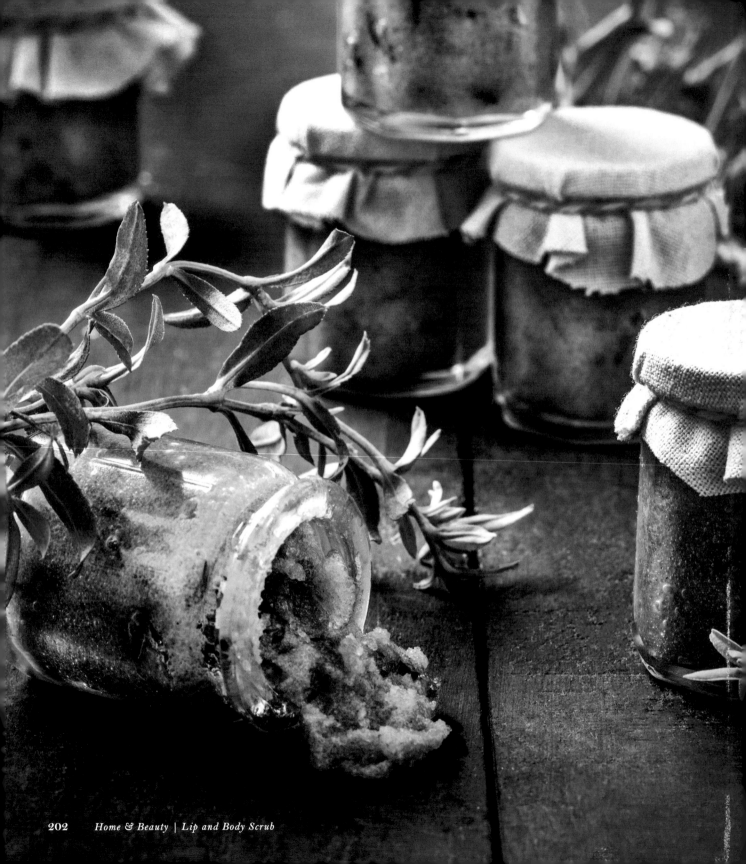

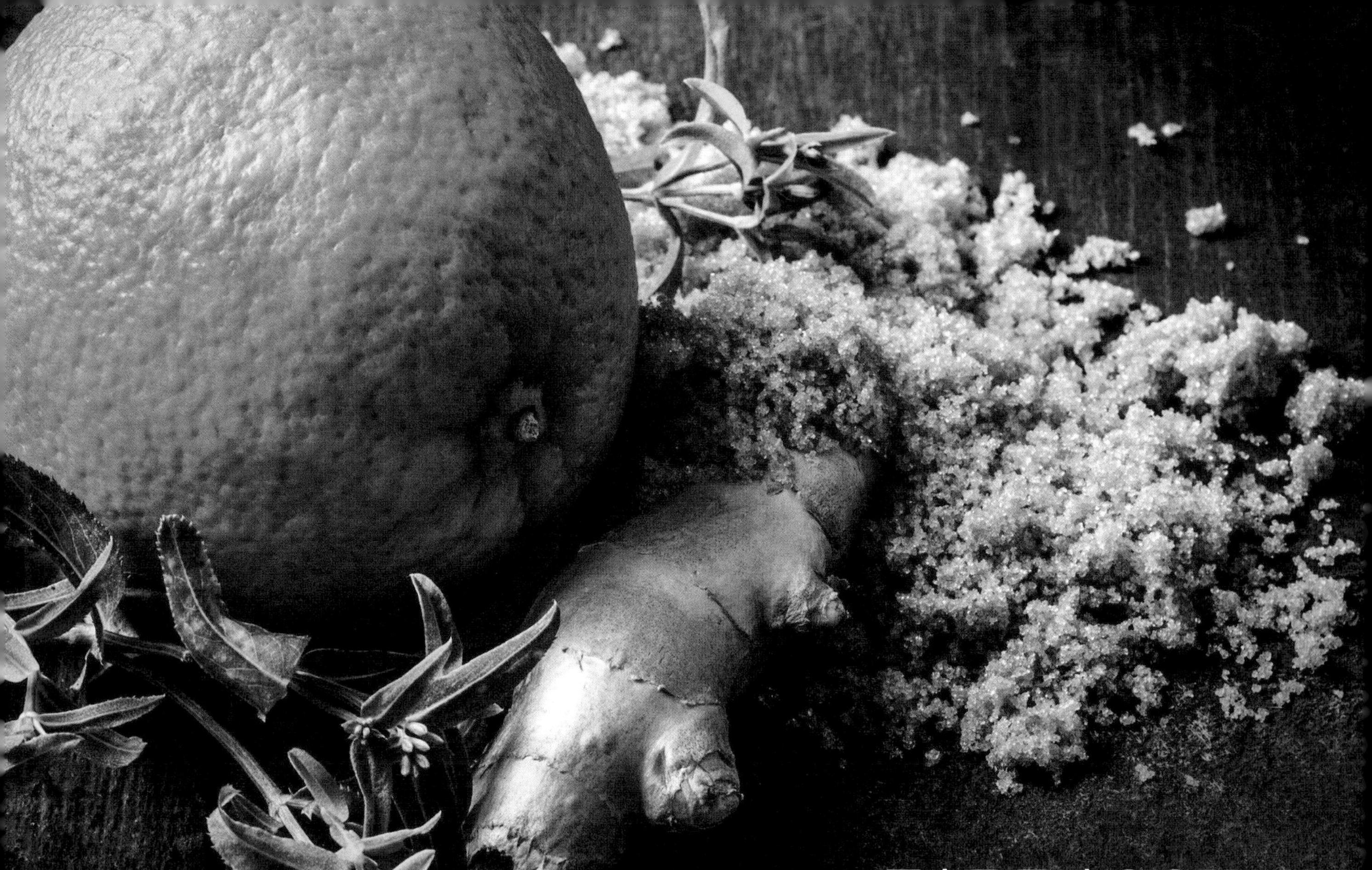

TARRAGON, ORANGE, & GINGER EXFOLIATING SUGAR LIP AND BODY SCRUB

Soothe tensed muscles and lift your mood while you buff your skin with a warm, spicy, and tangy sugar-scrub blend. The scrub is gentle enough for your lips but is also strong enough that it can be used all over the body.

1 cup brown sugar

3 Tbsp. coconut oil

5 drops orange essential oil, optional

2 drops ginger essential oil, optional

1 Tbsp. ground ginger

Zest of 2 oranges

3 sprigs fresh tarragon

¼ tsp. cinnamon

5 drops vitamin E oil

1. Collect leaves from the tarragon sprigs and muddle or chop finely.

2. Mix all the ingredients together.

3. Store in airtight container.

4. Refrigerate up to one week.

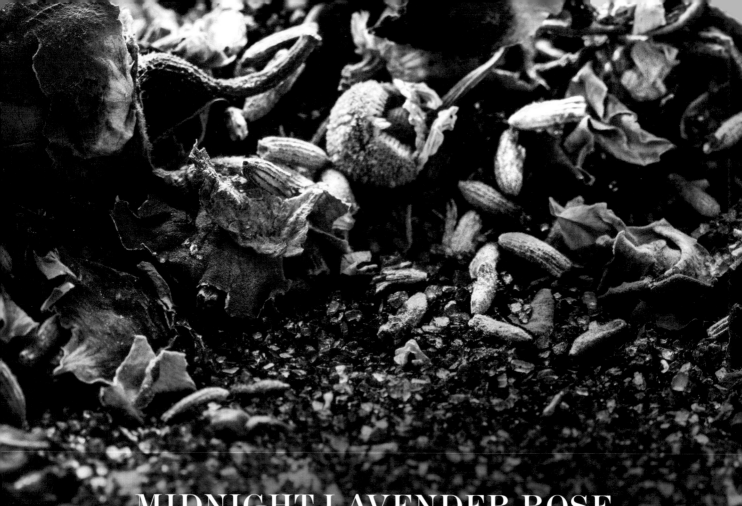

MIDNIGHT LAVENDER ROSE CHAMOMILE BATH SALTS

Relax with an evening bath, surrounded by the scents of lavender, chamomile, and rose. The lavender and chamomile are relaxing scents, and the rose adds sensuality. This bath salt heals and moisturizes too, making it great for all skin types.

1. Mix all the dry ingredients together.

2. Add the essential oils to the mixture. Stir.

3. Store in airtight container.

1 cup black sea salt

1 cup rose buds and/or rose petals

¼ cup lavender flowers

¼ cup chamomile

25 drops lavender essential oil

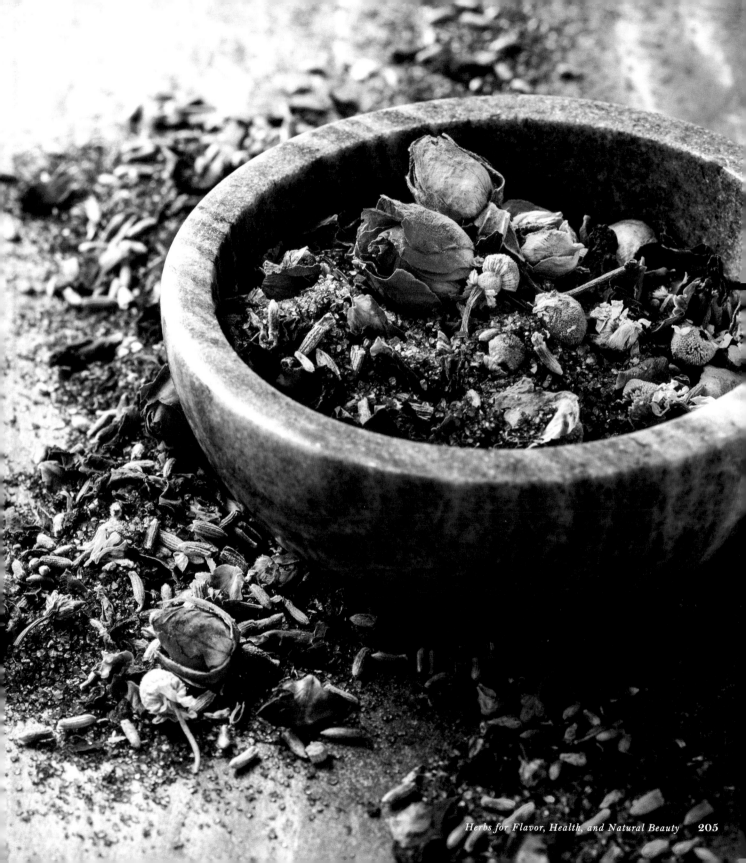

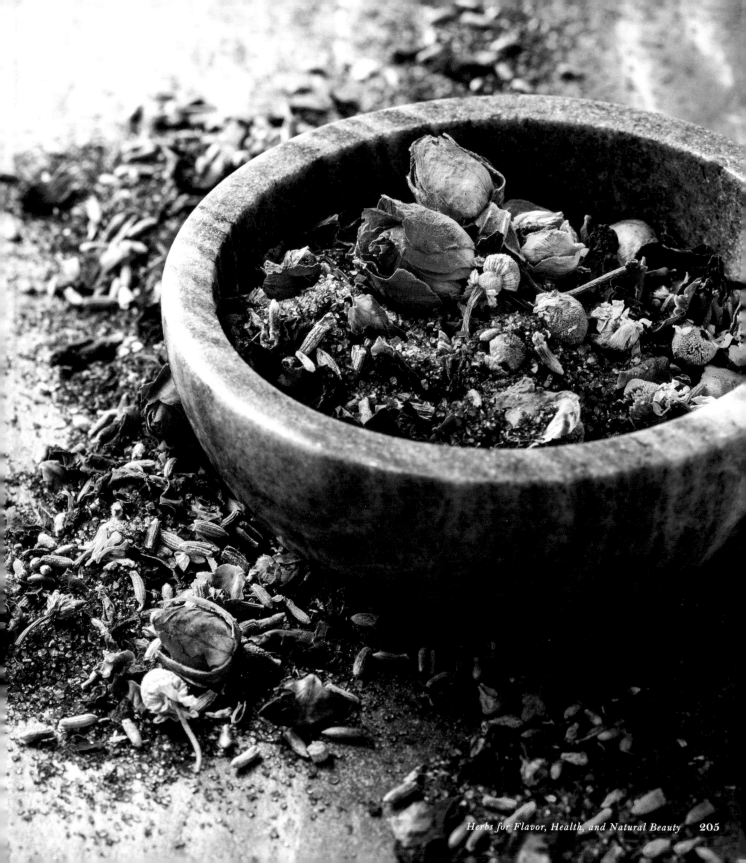

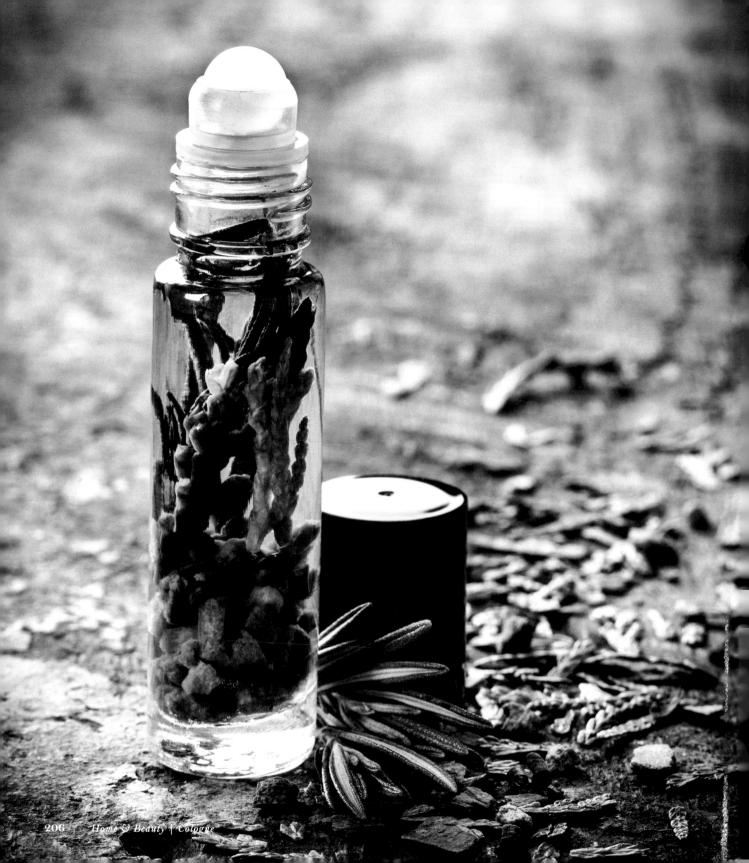

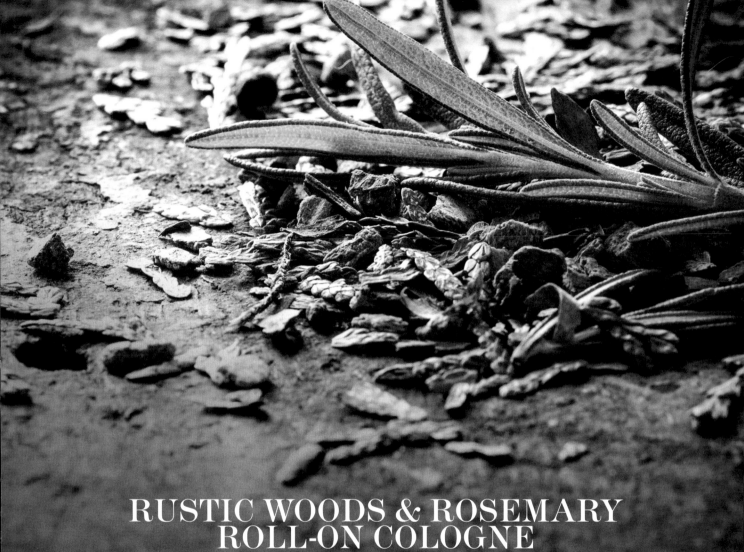

RUSTIC WOODS & ROSEMARY ROLL-ON COLOGNE

This natural, botanical scent slips easily onto the skin and compliments any mood. The romantic, citrus, and woodsy scent lasts for hours.

1. Add a few pieces of the dried cedar leaf, dried birch bark, and dried rosemary to the bottle (optional).

2. Add essential oils.

3. Fill the bottle to the top with vodka.

4. Store for one week to meld the scents.

Dried cedar leaf

Dried birch bark

Dried rosemary

BASE OILS:
4 drops cedar wood

4 drops rosemary

4 drops frankincense

MIDDLE TONES:
7 drops lavender

TOP NOTES:
7 drops sweet orange

.25 oz. vodka

1.25 oz. roll-on glass bottle

ENERGIZING MINT MOCHA LOOFAH SOAP

What better way to perk up in the morning than an energizing scent of mint coffee while you shower? This melt-and-pour mint-coffee soap uses coffee grounds and a natural loofah sponge for extra exfoliation.

3 cups shea melt and pour soap

¼ cup freshly ground high-quality coffee beans

¼ cup ground dried chocolate mint leaves

1 empty cleaned tube

1 spray bottle of rubbing alcohol to prevent bubbles

1 loofah sponge

Notes: Please use caution when handling melted soap. Do not put your hands directly into the hot soap. Use kitchen tongs or a long spoon handle to submerge the loofah.

1. Chop shea melt and pour soap into small chunks.

2. Place in a microwave-safe bowl and microwave for forty seconds. Stir and then continue to microwave in ten-second increments until melted.

3. Add coffee grounds and chocolate mint leaves. Stir.

4. Spray tube mold with rubbing alcohol.

5. Pour in soap mixture.

6. Submerge the loofah sponge in the mold, pressing into the soap mixture.

7. Spray with rubbing alcohol.

8. Let cool and harden for 2–3 hours.

9. Carefully remove from mold and use a knife to slice into five bars.

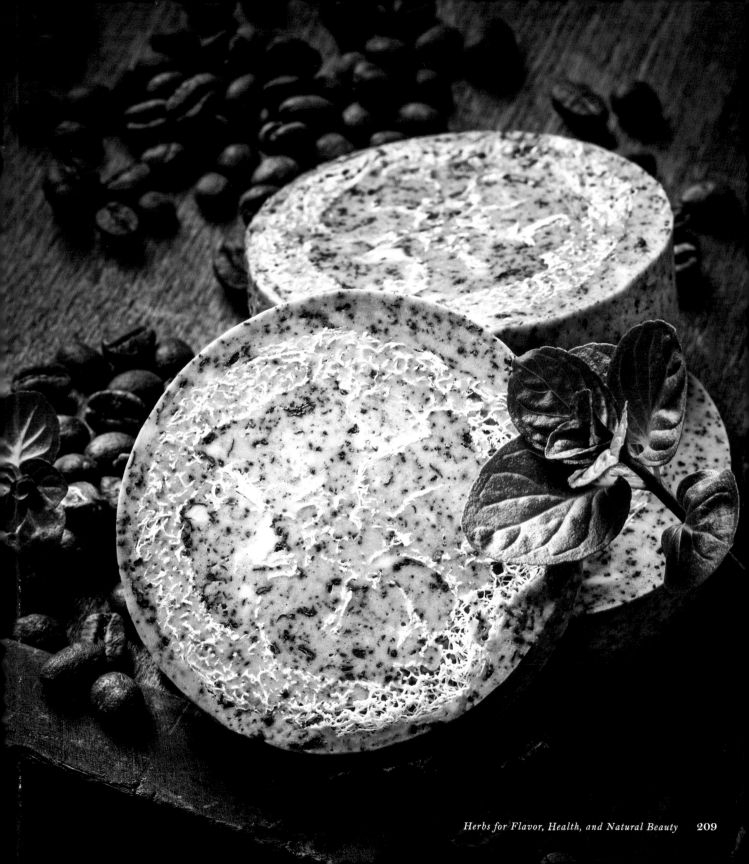

Herbs for Flavor, Health, and Natural Beauty

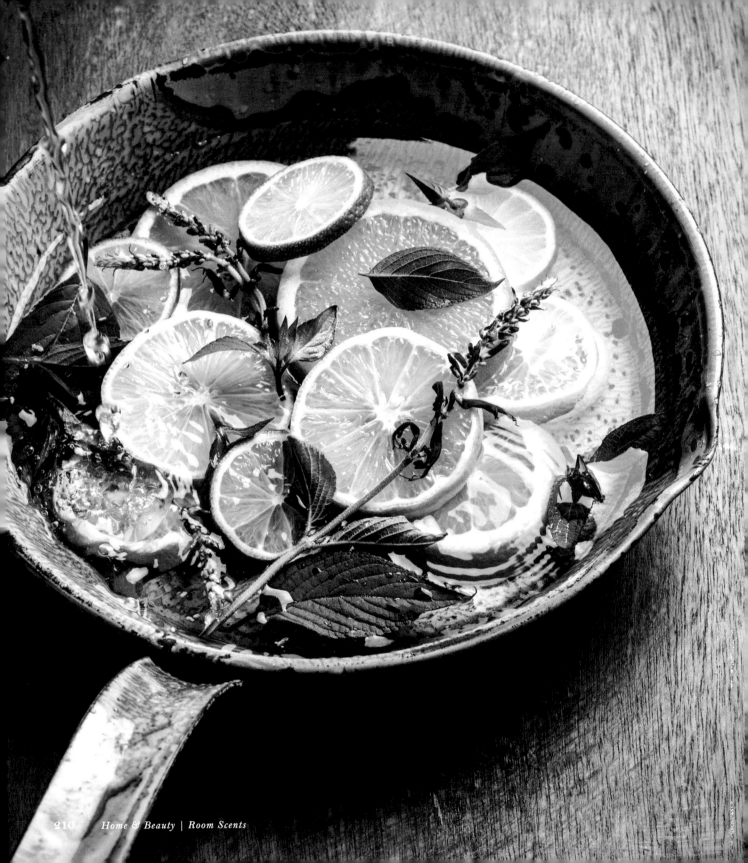

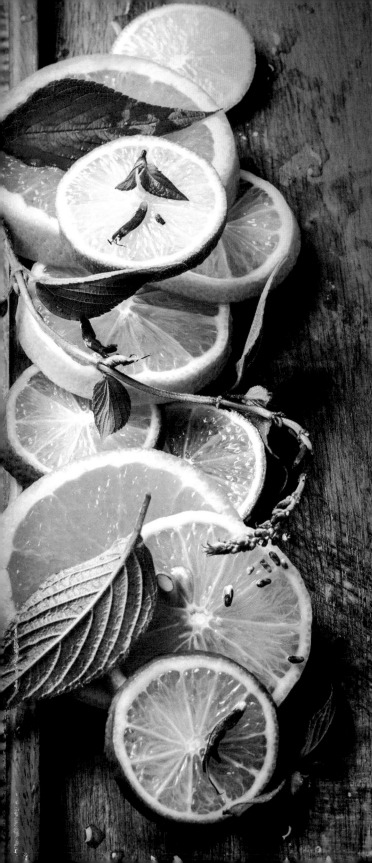

STOVETOP PINEAPPLE SAGE & CITRUS ROOM SCENTS

Heating aromatic ingredients over the stovetop is one truly simple way to add elegance and personality to your home. Pineapple sage is the secret to this tropical blend—a surefire way to liven up your spirit.

1 lime

1 orange

1 lemon

1 tsp. vanilla

Handful of pineapple sage

2 cups water

1 pot or pan

1. Slice fruit.

2. Add the first five ingredients in a pot or pan and immerse in two cups water.

3. Simmer over stove being careful not to let the water run out.

WILDFLOWER & THYME POTPOURRI

Lavender, thyme, and sandalwood oils are known to stimulate the mind, strengthen memory and concentration, and can help calm the nerves. Create a lovely scent and add visual beauty with a potpourri from these rich aromas! You can dry the botanicals yourself or buy them pre-dried.

¼ cup thyme

¼ cup lavender

¼ cup cornflower

¼ cup red clover

¼ cup heather flowers

¼ cup red sandalwood

10 drops sandalwood essential oil

10 drops thyme essential oil

10 drops lavender essential oil

1. Mix all dry ingredients together in a bowl.

2. Add the essential oils.

3. When scent wears down, you can apply desired amount of essential oils again.

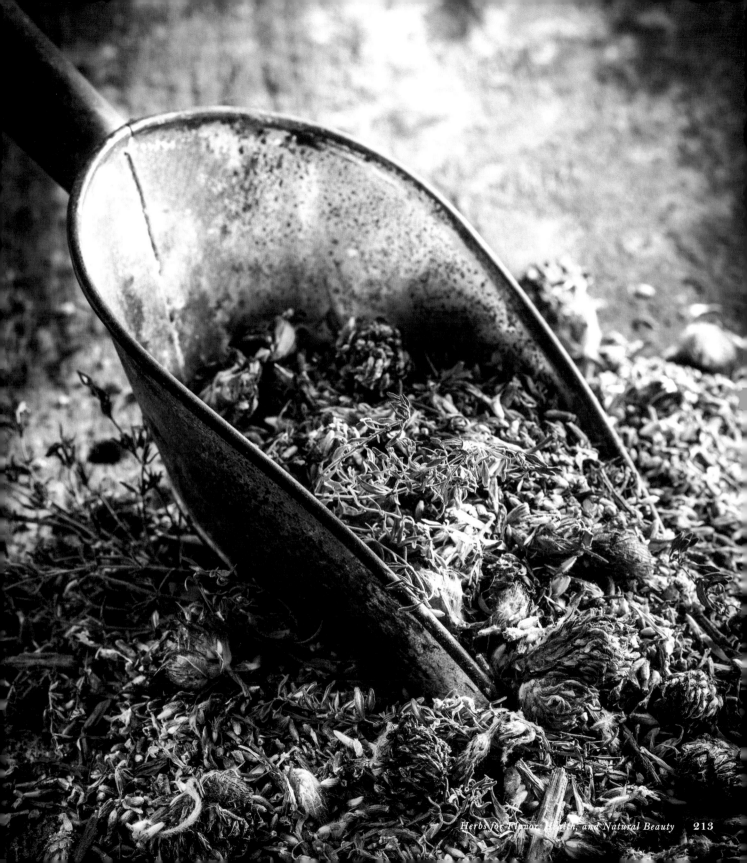

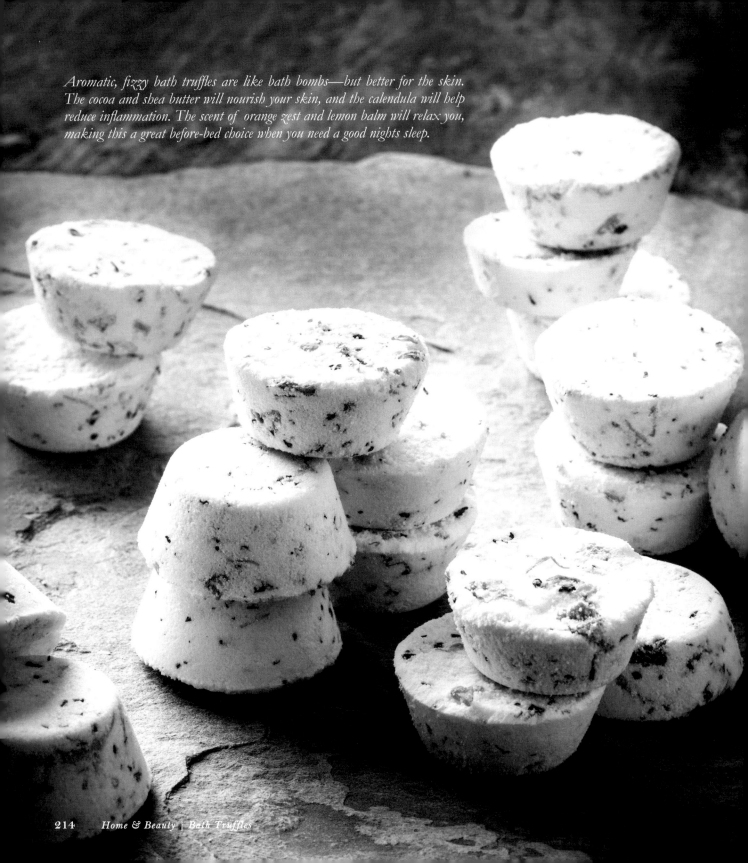

Aromatic, fizzy bath truffles are like bath bombs—but better for the skin. The cocoa and shea butter will nourish your skin, and the calendula will help reduce inflammation. The scent of orange zest and lemon balm will relax you, making this a great before-bed choice when you need a good nights sleep.

ZESTY ORANGE, CALENDULA, & LEMON BALM FIZZY BATH TRUFFLES

2½ cups baking soda

1¼ cup citric acid

¼ cup cocoa butter

¼ cup shea butter

5 drops sweet orange essential oil, optional

5 drops lemon essential oil, optional

2 Tbsp. orange zest

2 Tbsp. dried lemon balm

2 Tbsp. dried calendula

Rubber gloves

Molds (We used a mini muffin pan)

1. Wear gloves throughout the whole process.

2. Mix together the baking soda and citric acid. Set aside.

3. In a microwave-safe container, heat the cocoa butter and shea butter in the microwave for thirty seconds, stir and repeat the process in ten-second increments until it is in liquid form. Be sure to handle with care, as this will be hot.

4. Add essential oils if desired.

5. Slowly pour oil over the baking soda mixture while mixing with your hands until it feels like damp sand.

6. Add the orange zest, lemon balm, and dried calendula. Mix together.

7. Firmly pack the mix into molds.

8. Let dry for 24 hours.

This recipe makes about 24 mini muffin size truffles.

Note: Take caution when making the truffles, as the oils and butter may cause the tube molds to be slippery.

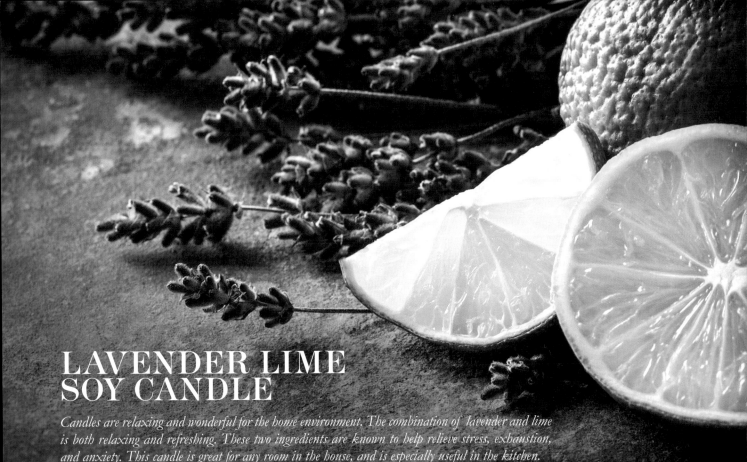

LAVENDER LIME SOY CANDLE

Candles are relaxing and wonderful for the home environment. The combination of lavender and lime is both relaxing and refreshing. These two ingredients are known to help relieve stress, exhaustion, and anxiety. This candle is great for any room in the house, and is especially useful in the kitchen.

1. Melt 3½ cups of soy chips in a double broiler.

2. Take off the heat. Dip the end of the wooden wick in the wax and adhere to the center of the bottom of the glass jar.

3. Add the essential oils. Fifteen drops of lavender and twenty-five drops of lime.

4. Let the candles set for twenty-four hours.

5. There may be dips in the center or cracks. Melt the remaining wax.

6. Take off heat and add remaining five drops each of lavender and lime essential oil. Pour over candle.

7. Let set for eight hours.

4½ cups soy chips

1 3-cup glass jar with a 2½- to 3-inch opening

20 drops of lavender essential oil

30 drops of lime essential oil

This recipe makes one candle.

Notes:

1. *If you do not care about the crack and dips, you can skip steps 6–8 and use all of the materials in steps 1–4.*

2. *Take caution when handling the candle wax, as it may be quite hot. Use tongs and gloves throughout the process.*

3. *Never leave a burning candle unattended.*

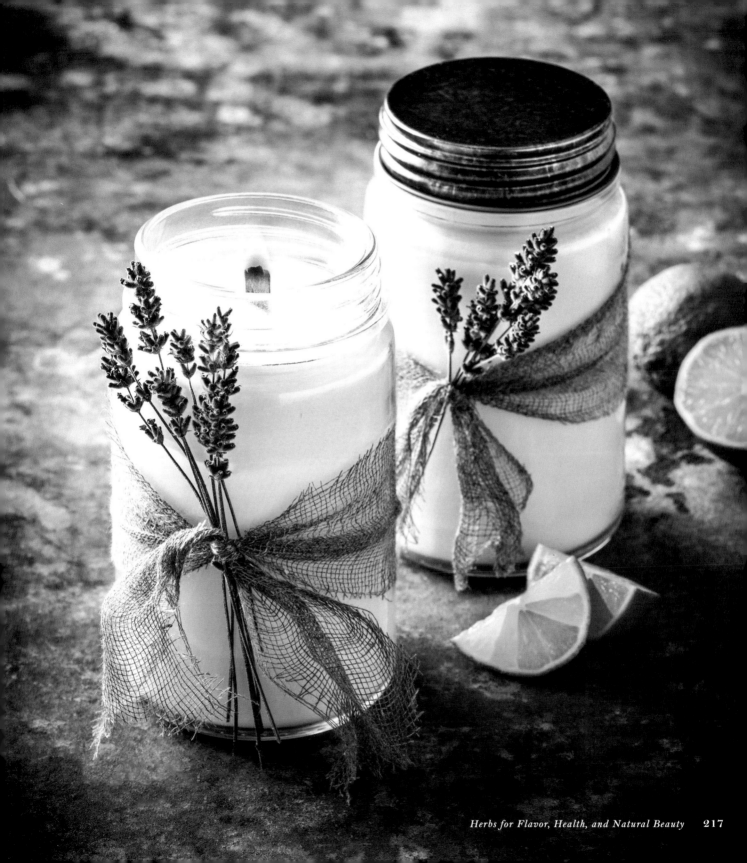

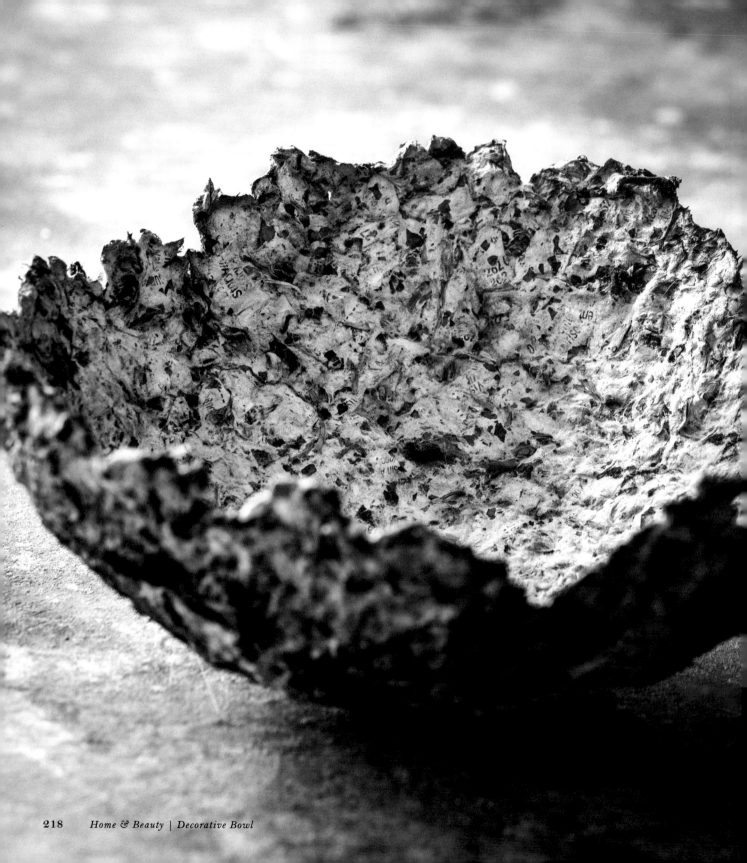

BOTANICAL RECYCLED PAPER DECORATIVE BOWLS

This sweet and delicate bowl also makes a great catch-all dish for small, loose items such as jewelry, spare change, or hairpins.

1. Tear or cut the paper into small pieces and put into a blender with water. Blend until the mixture becomes a rough pulp.

2. Add the rose petals, cornflower, calendula, lavender, and choice of dried green herb.

3. Pulse three times to mix together.

4. Add mixture to strainer over the sink.

5. Spread mixture over the entire mesh strainer and press to take out excess water.

6. Let dry.

7. Carefully peel away from strainer.

8. Spray with varnish in a well-ventilated area.

This recipe makes two 6-inch bowls.

Recycled paper
(We used newsprint)

2 cups warm water

¼ cup rose petals

¼ cup cornflower

¼ cup calendula

¼ cup lavender

¼ any dried green herb
(We used cilantro leaf because it still had a rich color after being dried)

1–2 metal mesh strainer(s), about 6 inches wide

SIMPLE MINT BEESWAX LIP BALM

Cool your lips with mint while healing them with a combination of coconut, beeswax and shea butter. Makes 8 ½-ounce tins.

2 Tbsp. mint-infused coconut oil, (see step 1 for directions)

2 Tbsp. beeswax

2 Tbsp. shea butter

15 drops peppermint essential oil

8½ oz. metal lip balm tins

1. To make mint-infused coconut oil, infuse one handful of mint leaves into ⅓ cup coconut oil for five hours in a double broiler. Strain. (You may have leftovers.)

2. Melt beeswax, shea butter, and two tablespoons infused coconut oil in a double broiler until melted. Stir frequently.

3. Turn off heat and remove from heat stove.

4. Add in essential oil and stir.

5. Pour in tins and wait until cool to cap.

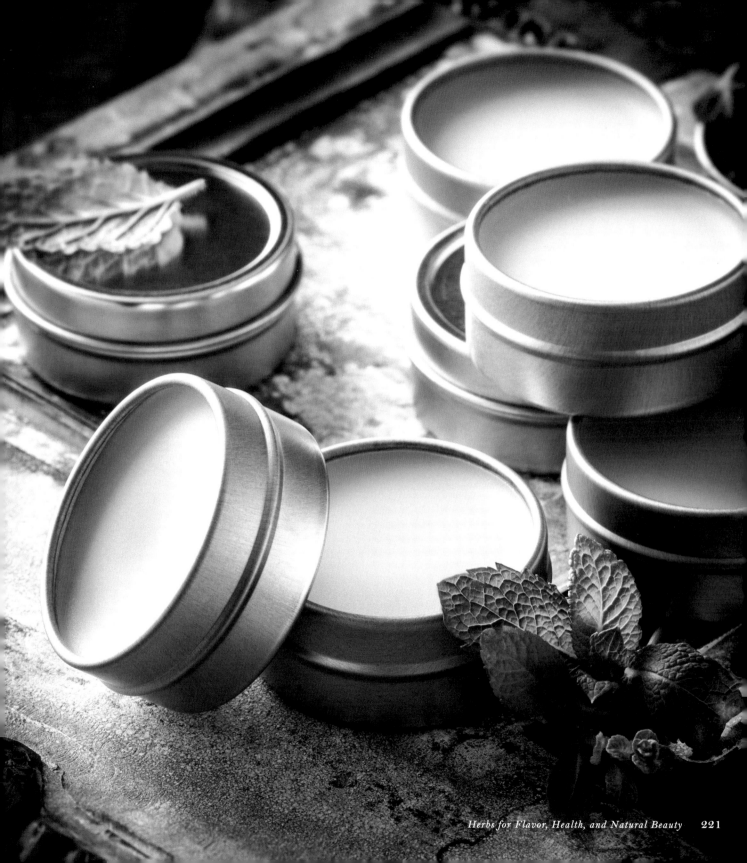

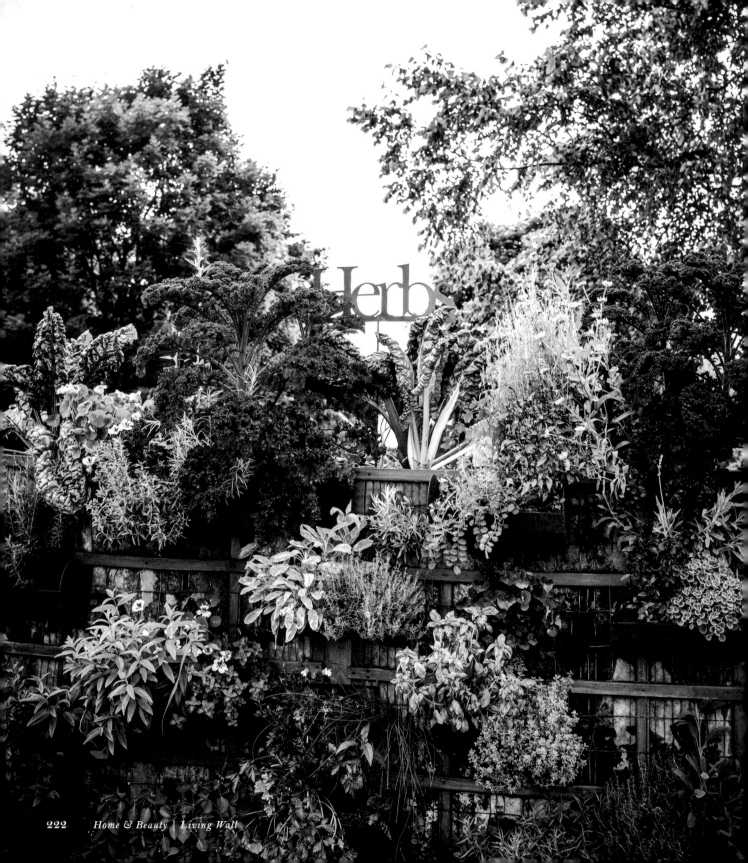

LIVING WALL

*H*aving an herb garden can sometimes be difficult. It usually requires a fair amount of physical space. If you live in a metropolitan area, having an herb garden in anything other than pots isn't really an option. Herb gardens can be prone to attacks from animals like rabbits, who love to feast on the fruits of your labor. It's enough to keep people from starting any kind of garden at all. There are options however, which can remedy a few of these issues, while also creating something beautiful as well. It's called a living wall. A living wall is basically a three-sided raised bed turned upright with plywood on one side and chicken wire and landscaping fabric on the other to keep in the dirt. Fasten this raised bed wall to permanent 4- x 4-inch posts that are cemented into the ground. This prevents the bed from getting blown over by wind gusts. The top is left open to allow for a way of adding the soil. It also creates an open planter on top where more herbs or vegetables can be added. A lightweight mixture with perlite, peat, and topsoil in the wall will keep the mixture from adding stress on the front or back. Holes are then cut in the chicken wire and fabric to allow for small herbs to be planted. Watering can be simplified by adding an easy drip irrigation or sprinkler system, which is available at most big box hardware stores or online.

The first living wall I made was not perfect. I realized that the dirt inside would settle, causing the plants near the top to lose dirt and moisture, while the plants on the bottom had too much weight because the water would filter down, causing them to get waterlogged. Also, the soil was not as rich the second year, and the dead annuals were difficult to remove because the roots needed to be pulled out of a small hole. It was fine for some herbs that were hearty like parsley, chives, and even tarragon, but basil, rosemary, and cuban oregano didn't do as well in the wall.

The solution was to add hanging planters on the outside of the wall, as seen in this photo. They allowed annuals like basil to be easily removed in the fall or following spring, while herbs like tarragon and parsley did just fine in the wall itself because they were perennials.

You can plant as many as 35–40 different herbs, edible flowers or even vegetables using an 8- x 5-inch wall like this one. By going vertical, it is easier to maintain and allows for the harvesting of herbs while standing, instead of bending down to cut them. Feel free to use these photos as inspiration for your own ideas.

Index

Index

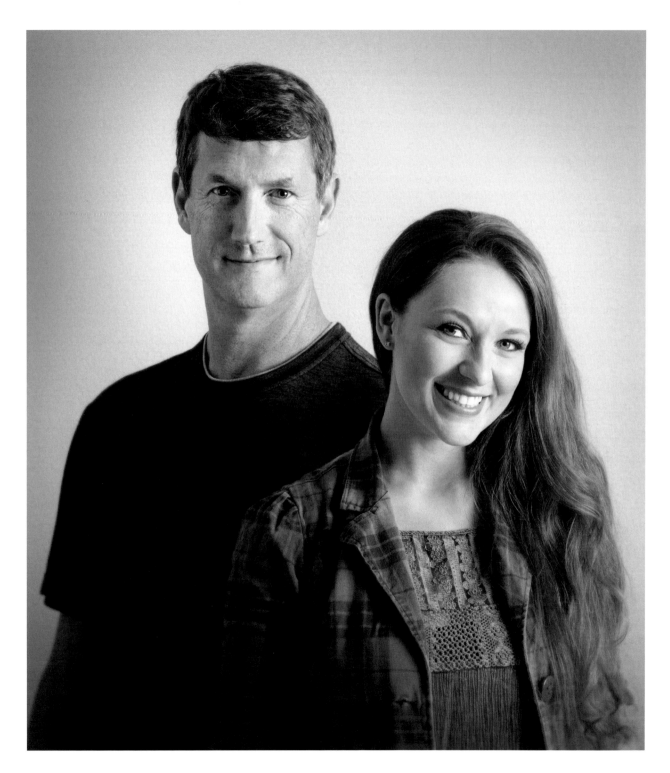

About the Authors

About the Authors

*J*ena and Jim started their blogging lives together almost four years ago, in January of 2013. Since then, they have collaborated on their award-winning blog, Little Rusted Ladle, creating mouthwatering images, tasty recipes, and home decor from food, flowers, herbs, and other products of nature. This is not how the story began with them, however.

Jena Weller Carlin grew up on an organic dairy farm in rural Wisconsin. She graduated from the University of Wisconsin-Stout, earning a Bachelor of Fine Arts degree with a major in painting and minor in photography. During college, she met her ever-supportive husband, Brandon Carlin. They moved to Milwaukee where Jena started her photography career working for Taste of Home Magazine. Here is where she started nurturing her love for food photography.

"There is something about capturing a still image and being able to smell it and feel its warmth. Food as a photography subject welds my urge for buying antique home goods and my creative nature for making imagery." This is how Jena describes her specialty. With her son, Austin, and another baby Carlin on the way, Jena enjoys all the spoils associated with having a loving family and a successful career.

Jim's food career began at culinary school where his passion for cooking came alive. After graduating from Blackhawk Technical College with a culinary arts degree, Jim worked as a cook and then as a chef at a number of restaurants in southern Wisconsin. While working at a country club, Jim was exposed to the world of food styling. Falling in love with the trade, he moved to Milwaukee where he worked as a freelance food stylist and recipe developer. His clients included dozens of companies such as Sara Lee, Kraft, and Taste of Home Magazine, where he met Jena.

It would be years later that he and Jena would meet again, and fate would lead them down the road they are on now. Jim currently lives in Janesville, Wisconsin where he enjoys his life as a single father of two grown children, Logan and Kennedy. He is still styling food and creating recipes after twenty-five years. Jim's philosophies about food are simple: "Nothing creates memories better than good food. When you create food that your friends and family love, you give them a little piece of yourself, something that they will always remember."

Visit them at:

www.jenacarlincreative.com   www.littlerustedladle.com   www.rudeonfood.com

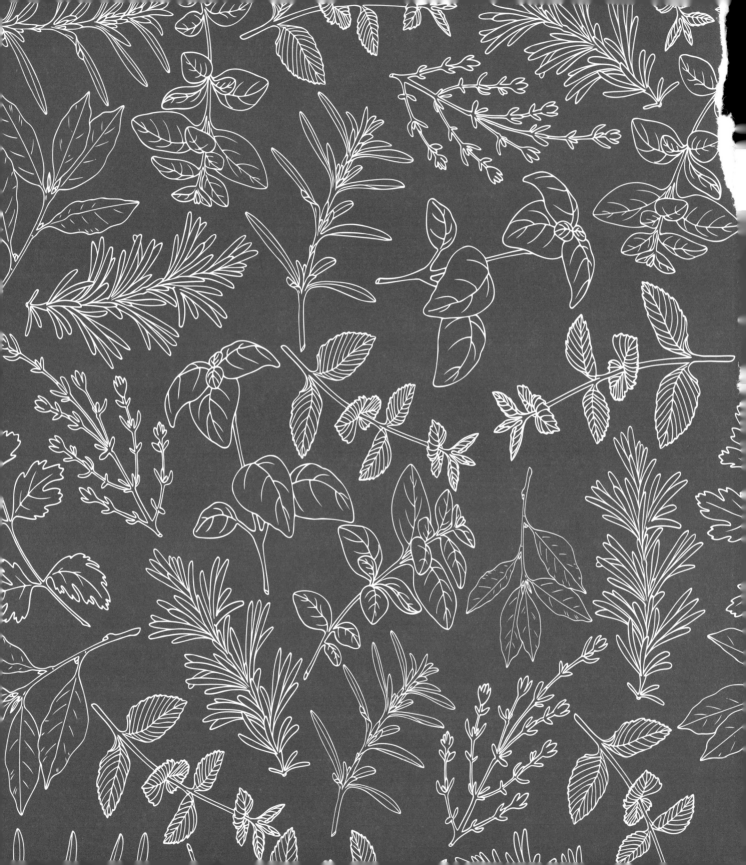